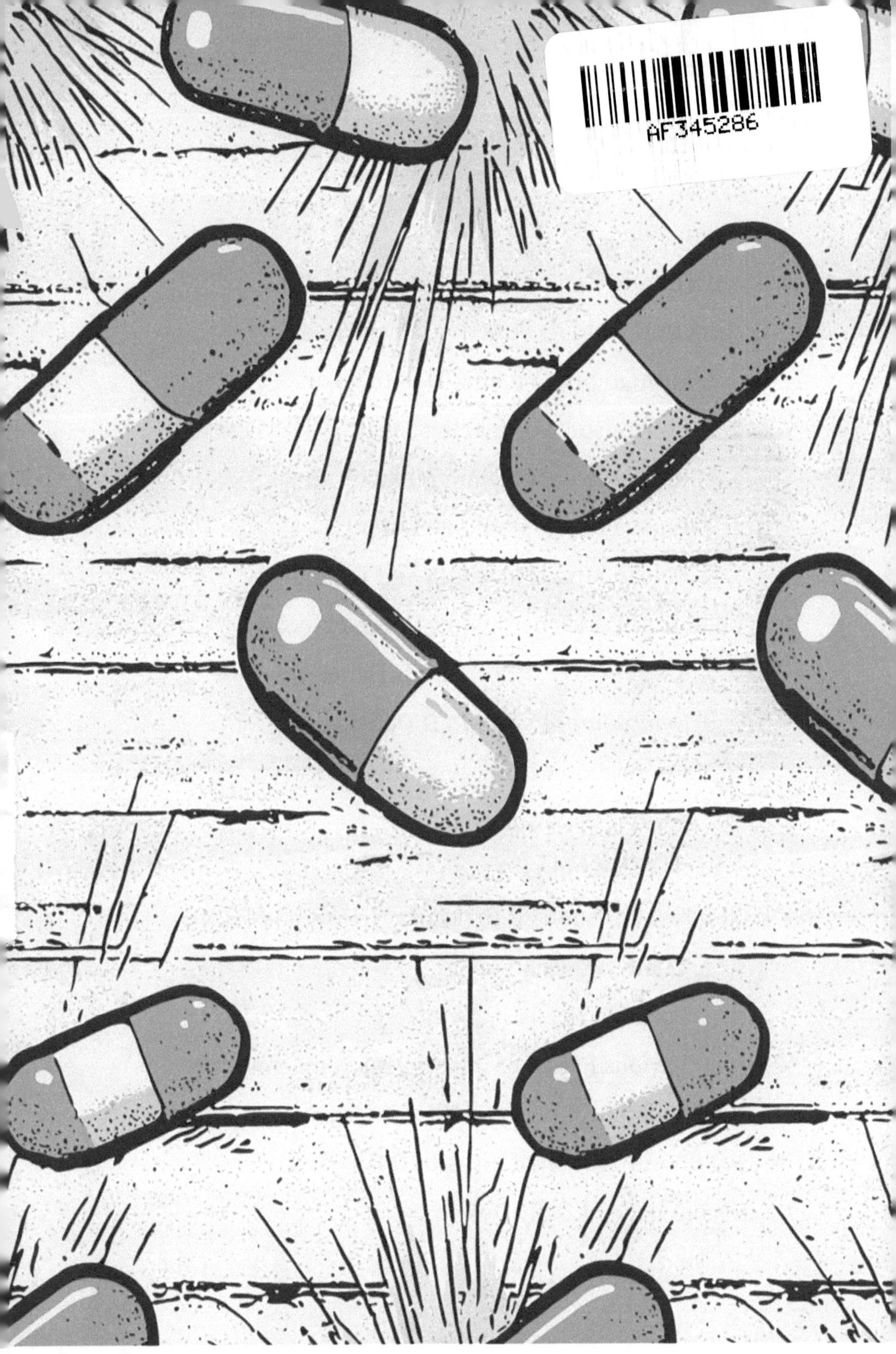

AF345286
AF345286

Table of Contents

Artemis Saage

Vitamin D3 Supplementation: The Essential Guide to High Dose Vitamin D3

Understanding Vitamin D Deficiency, Dosage Guidelines, and Health Benefits for Optimal Immune System and Bone Health

178 Sources
13 Photos / Graphics
21 Illustrations

Imprint

Saage Media GmbH
c/o SpinLab – The HHL Accelerator
Spinnereistraße 7
04179 Leipzig, Germany
E-Mail: contact@SaageMedia.com
Web: SaageMedia.com
Commercial Register: Local Court Leipzig, HRB 42755 (Handelsregister: Amtsgericht Leipzig, HRB 42755)
Managing Director: Rico Saage (Geschäftsführer)
VAT ID Number: DE369527893 (USt-IdNr.)

Publisher: Saage Media GmbH
Publication: 12.2024
Cover Design: Saage Media GmbH
ISBN Softcover: 978-3-384-45198-9
ISBN Ebook: 978-3-384-45199-6

Dear readers,

I sincerely thank you for choosing this book. With your choice, you have not only given me your trust but also a part of your valuable time. I truly appreciate that.

Vitamin D3 - the underestimated key to a strong immune system and healthy bones. Recent research shows that a large portion of the population has suboptimal vitamin D levels, with far-reaching consequences for health and well-being. This comprehensive specialist book imparts current expert knowledge on targeted vitamin D3 supplementation and its diverse effects on the body. You will learn how to determine your personal vitamin D needs, find the right dosage, and safely integrate supplementation into your daily routine. From its significance for the immune system to optimal absorption - here you will find scientifically grounded answers to all important questions regarding vitamin D3 supply. This book offers a practical guide for the safe and effective use of high-dose vitamin D3, based on current research findings. Understand the central role of vitamin D3 for your health and learn how targeted supplementation can sustainably improve your well-being.

I now wish you an inspiring and insightful reading experience. If you have any suggestions, criticism, or questions, I welcome your feedback. Only through active exchange with you, the readers, can future editions and works become even better. Stay curious!

Artemis Saage
Saage Media GmbH

- support@saagemedia.com
- Spinnereistraße 7 - c/o SpinLab – The HHL Accelerator, 04179 Leipzig, Germany

Introduction

To provide you with the best possible reading experience, we would like to familiarize you with the key features of this book. The chapters are arranged in a logical sequence, allowing you to read the book from beginning to end. At the same time, each chapter and subchapter has been designed as a standalone unit, so you can also selectively read specific sections that are of particular interest to you. Each chapter is based on careful research and includes comprehensive references throughout. All sources are directly linked, allowing you to delve deeper into the subject matter if interested. Images integrated into the text also include appropriate source citations and links. A complete overview of all sources and image credits can be found in the linked appendix. To effectively convey the most important information, each chapter concludes with a concise summary. Technical terms are underlined in the text and explained in a linked glossary placed directly below. For quick access to additional online content, you can scan the QR codes with your smartphone.

Additional bonus materials on our website
We provide the following exclusive materials on our website:

- Bonus content and additional chapters
- A compact overall summary
- A PDF file with all references
- Further reading recommendations

The website is currently under construction.

SaageBooks.com/vitamin_d3_supplementation-bonus-W81RER

1. Basics of Vitamin D3 Supplementation

The significance of Vitamin D3 for our health is becoming increasingly evident in medical research. What was once primarily associated with bone health is increasingly revealing itself as a versatile regulator of numerous bodily functions. But how exactly is Vitamin D3 produced and activated in our bodies? What role does it play in the regulation of the immune system? And why do so many people suffer from a deficiency despite the possibility of endogenous production? The complexity of Vitamin D3 supply becomes particularly apparent when considering the various influencing factors—from geographical location to individual lifestyle habits and genetic predispositions. Optimal supplementation therefore requires a fundamental understanding of the biochemical processes and their regulation in the body. This chapter systematically illuminates the scientific foundations of Vitamin D3 production and activation, as well as the various options for supplementation. Knowledge of these interconnections forms the basis for effective and individualized optimization of Vitamin D3 supply.

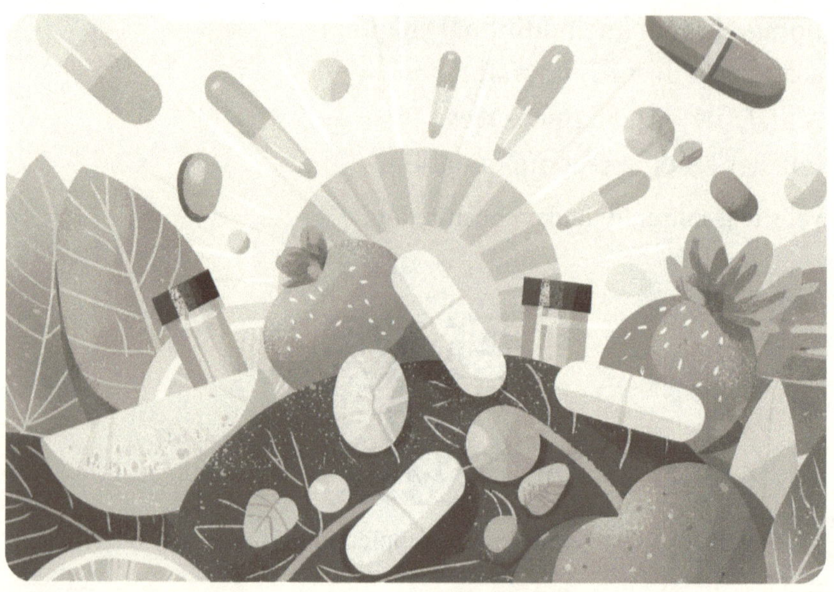

1. 1. Vitamin D3 and its Functions in the Body

he role of vitamin D3 in the human body is far more complex than long assumed. How does a single vitamin exert influence over such diverse processes as calcium metabolism, immune defense, and muscle strength? What occurs during the transformation from an initially inactive molecule to one of the most important hormones in our body? From its formation in the skin to its activation in various organs, vitamin D3 undergoes remarkable transformations. It not only regulates calcium balance but also influences the expression of hundreds of genes. The discovery of vitamin D receptors in nearly all body cells has fundamentally expanded our understanding of its diverse functions. The following sections illuminate the fascinating biochemical processes and demonstrate why optimal vitamin D3 supply is so significant for our health.

„Without vitamin D, only 10-15% of the calcium absorbed from food can be utilized by the body; with sufficient vitamin D, this rate increases to 30-40%.“

1. 1. 1. Formation of Vitamin D in the Skin

he formation of Vitamin D in the skin is a fascinating biochemical process that is largely dependent on sunlight exposure. When UVB rays hit our skin, a complex chain of reactions is initiated [s1]. In the epidermis, the outermost layer of skin, the molecule 7-dehydrocholesterol (7-DHC) is converted into previtamin D3 through the action of UVB radiation [s2]. However, this initial conversion is only the first step. The formed previtamin D3 is subsequently converted into vitamin D3 through a thermal process [s3]. From there, it enters the bloodstream, where it undergoes further transformations. In the liver, it is first converted to 25-hydroxyvitamin D3 (calcidiol) hydroxylated, the main form of vitamin D in the blood. The final activation occurs in the kidneys, where it is converted to 1,25-dihydroxyvitamin D3 (calcitriol) - the biologically active form [s4]. The efficiency of vitamin D formation is influenced by various factors. A particularly important factor is geographic location. People living at higher latitudes can produce virtually no vitamin D in their skin during the winter months - a phenomenon referred to as "vitamin D winter" [s3]. In Germany, for example, effective vitamin D synthesis is primarily possible from March to October, with the optimal time being between 10:00 AM and 4:00 PM [s5]. Skin pigmentation also plays a crucial role. Individuals with darker skin (skin type VI) require about five times longer than those with very light skin (skin type I) to produce the same amount of vitamin D [s5]. For instance, to produce 1000 IU of vitamin D, a person with skin type I needs about 5 minutes, while someone with skin type VI requires about 25 minutes. Age significantly affects vitamin D formation as well. Older individuals often have a reduced ability to synthesize vitamin D, as their skin contains less 7-DHC [s4]. This makes them particularly susceptible to vitamin D deficiency. For practical application, this means: moderate sun exposure of 10-15 minutes, two to three times a week, is usually sufficient to optimize vitamin D production [s6]. However, one should be cautious, as the same UVB rays responsible for vitamin D production can also cause sunburn and skin damage. Interestingly, skin cells (keratinocytes) themselves have the ability to locally activate and utilize vitamin D [s4]. This is important for various skin functions such as cell growth, wound healing, and maintaining the skin barrier. For individuals who spend a lot of time indoors or live in northern regions, vitamin D supplementation during the winter months may be advisable [s3].

Additionally, people with darker skin, older adults, and those who must avoid sunlight for health reasons should monitor their vitamin D levels. While the use of sunscreen theoretically affects vitamin D production, normal application does not lead to deficiency [s6]. A balanced approach is important here: after a brief, unprotected sun exposure, sunscreen should be applied to protect the skin from damage.

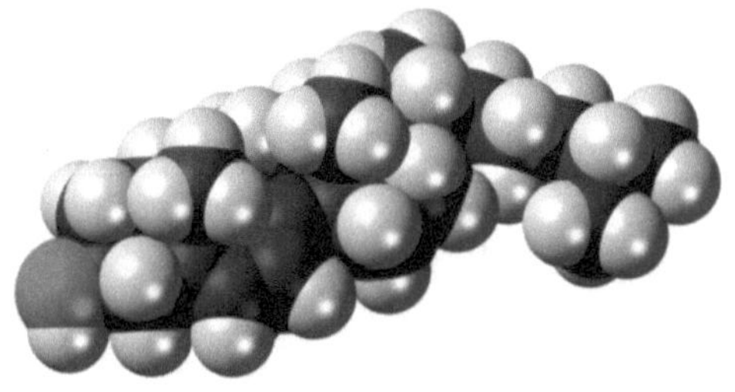

7-dehydrocholesterol [i1]

Glossary

Calcidiol

Storage form of vitamin D in the body, measured to determine vitamin D status in the blood.

Calcitriol

Hormone-like form of vitamin D that can directly bind to vitamin D receptors in various body cells.

Epidermis

The outermost layer of skin, which completely renews itself approximately every 4 weeks and consists of several layers of cells.

Hydroxylation

A chemical reaction in which a hydroxyl group (OH) is attached to a molecule, altering its properties.

Keratinocytes

Horn-forming cells that make up about 90% of all skin cells and are responsible for the formation of the stratum corneum.

1. 1. 2. Conversion to the Active Form

fter the intake of Vitamin D3, whether through sunlight exposure on the skin or dietary supplements, a complex activation process begins in the body. The initially inactive Vitamin D3 is stored in the body's fat cells, serving as a reserve for times of lower availability [s7]. This storage is particularly important for individuals in northern regions who are exposed to less sunlight during the winter months. The activation occurs in a precisely controlled two-step process. In the liver, a specific enzyme first converts Vitamin D3 into an intermediate form. Subsequently, another enzyme completes the conversion into the biologically active form [s8]. These enzymatic processes are highly efficient and have been optimized through evolutionary development [s9]. Of particular interest is the regulation of these conversion processes: The production of active Vitamin D3 in the kidneys is precisely controlled by various factors such as parathyroid hormone, calcium, phosphate, and FGF23 [s10]. This allows the body to adjust Vitamin D activation to its current needs. For example, if you have a low calcium level, more active Vitamin D is produced to enhance calcium absorption in the intestines. The active form, 1,25-dihydroxyvitamin D3, performs various functions in the body. A primary function is the regulation of calcium levels in the blood [s11]. It acts like a conductor, coordinating various processes: it increases calcium absorption in the intestines and can mobilize calcium from the bones when necessary. Particularly fascinating is the discovery that activated immune cells (macrophages) are also capable of locally activating Vitamin D [s11]. This explains the important role of Vitamin D for our immune system. For instance, when dealing with an infection, these cells can specifically produce active Vitamin D to support the immune response. The mechanism of action of active Vitamin D3 is complex and is based on epigenetic mechanisms. The hormone binds to its receptor (VDR) and influences gene expression by interacting with various proteins such as histone acetyltransferases [s12]. These molecular processes explain why Vitamin D can exert such diverse effects in the body—from bone health to immune regulation. Interestingly, an alternative metabolic pathway has also been discovered, leading to the formation of various hydroxymetabolites [s8]. These metabolites can also exhibit biological activities and expand the spectrum of Vitamin D effects in the body. For practical application, this means: Adequate Vitamin D supply is important for the body to have enough raw material for activation. It should be noted that the activation processes require time—one reason why regular intake is more important than sporadic high doses when supplementing. Additionally, certain diseases or medications may influence activation. In such cases, consulting a physician is particularly important to determine the optimal dosage. The efficiency of the conversion has significantly improved in recent decades due to new insights into the involved enzymes and microbial strains [s9]. This has also implications for the development of new therapeutic approaches for various diseases.

Glossary

Epigenetic
Heritable changes in gene activity that do not involve changes to the DNA sequence.

Histone Acetyltransferase
Enzymes that attach chemical markers to DNA packaging proteins, thereby influencing gene activity.

Macrophage
Immune cells that can engulf and destroy pathogens.

Parathyroid Hormone
A hormone produced by the parathyroid glands that regulates calcium and phosphate balance and works closely with Vitamin D.

1. 1. 3. Regulation of Calcium Metabolism

he regulation of calcium metabolism is a highly complex system in which vitamin D3 plays a central role. This vital process ensures that the calcium level in the blood is maintained within a very narrow range, which is essential for numerous bodily functions [s13]. A fascinating aspect is the efficiency of calcium absorption in the intestine: Without vitamin D, only 10-15% of the calcium ingested through food can be utilized by the body. With sufficient vitamin D, this rate increases to an impressive 30-40% [s13]. This underscores the importance of adequate vitamin D supply for individuals who rely on optimal calcium absorption—such as pregnant women, nursing mothers, or those at increased risk of osteoporosis. At the molecular level, the active form of vitamin D3 (1,25(OH)2D3) regulates every single step of calcium transport through the intestinal wall. This occurs through the activation of various proteins: The calcium channel TRPV6 facilitates absorption into the intestinal cells, the calcium-binding protein Calbindin-D9k transports calcium through the cell, and the calcium-ATPase PMCA1b ensures further transport into the blood [s14]. One can envision this process as a precisely choreographed ballet, where each step is perfectly coordinated with the others. The parathyroid glands also play an important role in this regulatory system. They produce the parathormon, which acts like a thermostat for calcium levels [s15]. When the calcium level in the blood drops, more parathyroid hormone is released. This leads to three important adjustments: 1. Increased calcium release from the bones 2. Enhanced calcium reabsorption in the kidneys 3. Increased vitamin D activation As one ages, this finely tuned system changes. The ability to absorb calcium in the intestine decreases, which is associated with a reduced expression of the necessary proteins (TRPV6 and Calbindin-D9k) [s14]. At the same time, the degradation rate of active vitamin D3 increases due to heightened activity of the enzyme CYP24A1 [s14]. This explains why older individuals are often affected by calcium and vitamin D deficiencies and consequently have an increased risk of osteoporosis.

Practical recommendations that can be derived from these findings:
- Pay particular attention to adequate calcium and vitamin D supply, especially in old age
- Consume calcium-rich meals preferably together with vitamin D-containing foods
- Consider that calcium absorption decreases with age and adjust your diet accordingly
- Regularly check your vitamin D and calcium levels, especially if you belong to a risk group

The significance of this precise regulation becomes particularly evident when one considers that calcium is not only important for healthy bones but is also required for muscle contraction, nerve signal transmission, and many other vital processes [s16]. A well-functioning calcium metabolism is thus fundamental to our health.

1. 1. 4. Impact on the Immune System

itamin D3 plays a central and fascinating role in the regulation of our immune system. Its mode of action is highly complex and occurs through various mechanisms that have only been fully understood in recent years [s17]. A particularly interesting aspect is the ability of Vitamin D3 to influence both the innate and adaptive immune systems. Immune cells contain specific Vitamin D receptors (VDR) and enzymes that enable the cells to process and utilize Vitamin D directly [s17]. This explains why individuals with a Vitamin D deficiency are more prone to infections—especially during the winter months when the body's own Vitamin D production is already reduced [s18]. The immunomodulatory effect of Vitamin D3 is particularly impressive in its ability to regulate approximately 900 different genes [s19]. A practical example: When you encounter a pathogen, Vitamin D3 supports your immune defense by promoting the production of antimicrobial peptides—the body's own "antibiotics" that can combat bacteria, viruses, and fungi [s19].

Notably, Vitamin D3 has a balancing effect on the immune system. It acts like a wise conductor, calming an overactive immune system while activating a weak one [s20]. This occurs, among other things, through:
- The promotion of regulatory T-cells that dampen excessive immune reactions
- The reduction of pro-inflammatory signaling molecules
- The increase of anti-inflammatory substances [s19]

For individuals with autoimmune diseases, it is particularly relevant that Vitamin D3 can inhibit the overreaction of the immune system [s20]. Studies have shown that a Vitamin D deficiency increases the risk of various autoimmune diseases [s18]. Interestingly, there are gender-specific differences: In women, the effect of Vitamin D3 seems to be enhanced by estrogen [s21].

Practical recommendations for daily life:
- Pay special attention to adequate Vitamin D supply, especially during the dark season
- If you experience frequent infections, have your Vitamin D levels checked
- Individuals with autoimmune diseases should regularly monitor their Vitamin D status
- Pregnant and breastfeeding mothers require special attention regarding their Vitamin D supply

The effect of Vitamin D3 on the immune system also extends to the <u>blood-brain barrier</u>, where it regulates the migration of immune cells [s22]. This is particularly important for neurological diseases such as multiple sclerosis, where a Vitamin D deficiency has been associated with an increased risk of disease [s23]. Remarkably, Vitamin D3 also plays a role in combating <u>oxidative stress</u> and improving barrier function in the respiratory tract [s19]. This explains why adequate Vitamin D supply is particularly important for the prevention of respiratory infections.

Antimicrobial Peptides

Small protein molecules that act like natural antibiotics and are part of the body's defense.

Blood-Brain Barrier

A natural barrier between blood vessels and brain tissue that keeps harmful substances away from the brain.

Immunomodulatory

Describes the ability of a substance to alter the activity of the immune system—it can either enhance or suppress it.

Oxidative Stress

A condition in which there are too many aggressive oxygen compounds in the body that can damage cells and tissues.

T-Cell

White blood cells that mature in the thymus and play a central role in targeted immune defense.

1. 1. 5. Role in Muscle Strength and Function

itamin D3 plays a crucial role in muscle strength and function, with its mechanisms being complex and multifaceted. In skeletal muscles, there are specific vitamin D receptors (VDR) that optimize muscle performance at various levels when adequately supplied [s24]. Of particular interest is the influence at the cellular level: Vitamin D3 activates genes that regulate muscle growth and differentiation. This is especially significant for fast-twitch muscle fibers (Type II fibers), which are responsible for explosive power development [s25]. The genomic effect includes promoting calcium availability in muscle cells as well as supporting muscle cell differentiation and proliferation [s26]. A fascinating aspect is the role of Vitamin D3 in mitochondrial function. Recent research shows that a deficiency impairs the oxidative capacity of skeletal muscles. The mitochondria, as the "powerhouses" of the cells, cannot function optimally with insufficient vitamin D supply, directly affecting energy provision and thus muscle strength [s27]. For athletes and active individuals, it is particularly relevant that Vitamin D3 can shorten recovery time after training. This occurs through the promotion of myogenic differentiation and proliferation, as well as the downregulation of myostatin [s28]. A practical example: Athletes with optimal vitamin D levels demonstrate better jumping ability, maximum oxygen uptake, and sprinting capacity [s24].

The effects of a vitamin D deficiency on muscle are extensive:
- Reduced muscle strength and performance
- Increased risk of muscle weakness and sarcopenia
- Prolonged recovery times after injuries
- Impaired insulin sensitivity of the muscles [s29]

Particularly interesting are the results of clinical studies: A high-dose vitamin D3 supplementation led to a 34% increase in serum levels and a 13% improvement in muscle strength within just 8 days [s30]. This demonstrates how quickly the body can respond to optimized supply.

For practical application, the following recommendations arise:
- Regular monitoring of vitamin D status, especially during intense physical activity
- Special attention during the winter months when the body's own production is reduced
- Adjustment of supplementation in case of increased demand (e.g., intense training)
- Consideration of individual factors such as skin type and training intensity

Research also shows an interesting connection between Vitamin D3 and testosterone production, which is relevant for muscle building [s28]. This explains why optimal vitamin D supply can be particularly important for strength athletes. For older individuals, the role of Vitamin D3 in muscle health is especially important. Supplementation can not only improve muscle strength but also reduce the risk of falls [s31]. This is particularly relevant for the prevention of age-related muscle loss and the maintenance of mobility in old age.

Glossary

Mitochondrion

Cell organelles that provide energy in the form of ATP for the cell through the metabolism of nutrients. A single muscle tissue can contain thousands of them.

Myogenic Differentiation

Developmental process in which immature muscle precursor cells develop into functional muscle cells. Important for muscle growth and regeneration.

Myostatin

A protein that naturally limits muscle growth. Its inhibition can lead to increased muscle development.

Sarcopenia

An age-related condition characterized by progressive loss of muscle mass, strength, and function. Primarily affects individuals over 60 years old.

Summary - 1. 1. Vitamin D3 and its Functions in the Body

- UVB radiation converts 7-dehydrocholesterol in the epidermis to previtamin D3.
- Individuals with skin type VI require approximately five times longer than those with skin type I for the same vitamin D production.
- Keratinocytes can locally activate vitamin D and utilize it for skin functions.
- The enzymatic activation occurs in a precisely controlled two-step process.
- Activated macrophages can locally activate vitamin D for immune functions.
- Vitamin D acts through epigenetic mechanisms by interacting with histone acetyltransferases.
- Without vitamin D, only 10-15% of dietary calcium can be utilized; with vitamin D, the rate increases to 30-40%.
- Calcium transport occurs via TRPV6 channels, Calbindin-D9k, and PMCA1b pumps.
- With age, the degradation rate of active vitamin D3 increases due to heightened CYP24A1 activity.
- Vitamin D3 regulates approximately 900 different genes in the immune system.
- Vitamin D3 promotes the production of endogenous antimicrobial peptides.
- Estrogen enhances the immunological effect of vitamin D3 in women.
- Vitamin D3 regulates the migration of immune cells at the blood-brain barrier.
- In skeletal muscles, vitamin D3 activates genes for growth and differentiation, particularly in type II fibers.
- High-dose supplementation resulted in a 34% increase in serum levels and 13% more muscle strength within 8 days.

1. 2. Vitamin D Deficiency and its Consequences

The significance of vitamin D for human health extends far beyond bone metabolism. But how does a vitamin D deficiency actually arise, and what consequences does it have for our organism? While over a billion people worldwide are affected by vitamin D deficiency, symptoms often remain unrecognized for a long time. Particularly in Europe, where about 40% of the population has insufficient vitamin D levels, the question of causes and health consequences arises. From bone health to the immune system and even mental well-being – the effects of a vitamin D deficiency can influence every aspect of our health. Recent scientific research has uncovered surprising connections that have fundamentally expanded our understanding of the role of this essential vitamin.

„Worldwide, over one billion people are affected by a vitamin D deficiency, with the prevalence in Europe being particularly high at around 40%.“

1. 2. 1. Risk Factors for Vitamin D Deficiency

vitamin D deficiency can be influenced by various risk factors, which can be lifestyle-related, genetic, or disease-related. Worldwide, over one billion people are affected by vitamin D deficiency [s32], with the prevalence in Europe being particularly high at about 40% [s33]. One of the main risk factors is insufficient sun exposure [s34]. Individuals who spend little time outdoors, such as those engaged in predominantly sedentary office work, are particularly at risk. A practical tip would be to schedule at least 15-20 minutes of walking during lunchtime each day, ideally with uncovered forearms and face. Geographical location also plays an important role [s35]. In higher latitudes, such as Northern and Central Europe, UVB radiation is often insufficient for adequate vitamin D production, especially during the winter months. People in these regions should pay increased attention to a vitamin D-rich diet and consider supplementation if necessary [s36]. Skin pigmentation is another significant factor [s37]. Individuals with darker skin require longer sun exposure to produce the same amount of vitamin D as those with lighter skin. Studies show that non-white individuals exhibit higher rates of vitamin D deficiency than European Caucasians [s33]. Certain life stages and circumstances significantly increase the risk of deficiency. Breastfeeding infants are particularly vulnerable, as breast milk alone does not provide sufficient vitamin D [s37]. Here, medically supervised supplementation is often necessary. Older adults also have an increased risk, as their skin is less efficient at producing vitamin D, and kidney function declines in activating the vitamin [s37]. Various diseases can also lead to vitamin D deficiency. In chronic kidney or liver diseases, the conversion of vitamin D to its active form is impaired [s34]. The prevalence among dialysis patients ranges from 85 to 99% [s33]. Individuals with inflammatory bowel diseases, celiac disease, or after bariatric surgery have an increased risk due to impaired absorption capacity [s34]. Obesity represents another important risk factor [s37]. Body fat binds vitamin D and prevents its absorption into the bloodstream. Therefore, individuals with excess weight should pay particular attention to their vitamin D levels and discuss tailored supplementation with their doctor if necessary. Certain medications can also influence vitamin D metabolism [s37]. These include some cholesterol-lowering drugs, antiepileptics, steroids, and weight loss medications. Patients taking these medications should regularly check their vitamin D levels. Cultural and lifestyle factors also play a role. Individuals who cover their skin largely for religious or cultural reasons, as well as those who consistently use sunscreen, have an increased risk of vitamin D deficiency [s35]. A balanced approach between sun protection and controlled sun exposure, such as short morning or late afternoon walks, could be beneficial. The consequences of vitamin D deficiency are far-reaching and can cause various health problems, from pregnancy complications to autoimmune diseases, as well as an increased risk of cardiovascular diseases and certain cancers [s32]. Therefore, individuals with risk factors should regularly check their vitamin D levels and consider targeted supplementation under medical supervision.

Glossary

Bariatric Surgery
> Surgical procedure for weight reduction by reducing the size of the stomach or rerouting the digestive tract, usually applied in cases of morbid obesity.

Celiac Disease
> Hereditary autoimmune disease in which the immune system reacts to gluten and damages the intestinal mucosa, potentially leading to nutrient deficiencies.

Obesity
> Medical term for severe overweight, where the body fat percentage is pathologically elevated, leading to health risks.

Prevalence
> Refers to the frequency of a disease or condition in a specific population group at a given time, expressed as the proportion of affected individuals to the total population.

1. 2. 2. Symptoms of Vitamin D Deficiency

vitamin D deficiency can manifest through a variety of symptoms, with interestingly, the majority of affected individuals initially showing no obvious complaints [s38]. This fact makes early detection particularly challenging and underscores the importance of regular health check-ups, especially for individuals with known risk factors. Characteristic symptoms primarily include complaints related to the musculoskeletal system. Scientific studies demonstrate a clear correlation between low vitamin D levels and adverse effects on bone health [s39]. This often manifests as diffuse bone pain, which affected individuals frequently describe as dull and deep-seated. These pains can be exacerbated, particularly in the morning after waking or during prolonged physical exertion. A practical tip for daily life is to pay attention to early warning signs such as recurring muscle and joint pain and not dismiss them as normal signs of aging. Bone substance can increasingly deteriorate with a prolonged deficiency, significantly raising the risk of fractures [s40]. This is particularly problematic for older individuals, who may already have an increased tendency to fall. Therefore, at-risk individuals should proactively adjust their living environment, for example, by installing grab bars in the bathroom or removing tripping hazards such as loose rugs. Another common symptom is pronounced muscle weakness, which is particularly noticeable when climbing stairs or rising from a squat. Affected individuals often report increased fatigue during everyday activities. To counteract this, gentle but regular strength training can be beneficial—however, the vitamin D status should be checked before starting any training program. Particularly concerning is the finding that severe vitamin D deficiency drastically increases the risk of excessive mortality and infections [s40]. This is especially evident in critically ill patients, where low vitamin D levels correlate with greater disease severity and mortality [s39]. Interestingly, there is also a connection in women with hypermobility disorders, who may have an increased risk for certain gynecological complaints [s41]. This underscores the complexity of the effects of vitamin D deficiency on various body systems. Symptoms can also manifest on a psychological level. Many affected individuals report mood swings and depressive symptoms, particularly during the darker months of the year. A regular daily rhythm with sufficient time spent outdoors can already show positive effects. Due to the often nonspecific symptomatology, it is important to consider a possible vitamin D deficiency in the case of persistent complaints such as chronic fatigue, muscle pain, or recurrent infections and to clarify this through a blood test. Early detection and treatment can help prevent serious secondary diseases. For self-monitoring, it is helpful to keep a symptom diary, documenting complaints, their intensity, and possible triggering factors. These records can provide valuable insights for the treating physician in making a diagnosis.

Glossary

hypermobility
Refers to excessive joint mobility that exceeds the normal range. It can be congenital or arise from certain connective tissue disorders.

1. 2. 3. Connection with Autoimmune Diseases

vitamin D deficiency is closely linked to the development and progression of various autoimmune diseases [s42]. Recent scientific research has shown that vitamin D is not only important for bone metabolism but also plays a central role in regulating the immune system [s43]. Particularly interesting is the gender-specific component: In women, the connection between vitamin D deficiency and autoimmune diseases appears to be particularly pronounced. This is partly due to the fact that estrogen enhances the effects of vitamin D and leads to a stronger anti-inflammatory response [s44]. This finding is especially relevant, as many autoimmune diseases occur more frequently in women. Concrete examples of the connection between vitamin D and autoimmune diseases can be found in various conditions: In multiple sclerosis (MS), it is evident that a vitamin D deficiency in childhood is considered a significant risk factor [s45]. Therefore, it is advisable for parents to ensure adequate vitamin D supply for their children, especially in the early years of life. This can be supported by regular outdoor activities and a balanced diet. In type 1 diabetes, a Finnish cohort study provides impressive results: Children who regularly supplemented vitamin D developed type 1 diabetes 80% less frequently [s45]. This underscores the importance of adequate vitamin D supply in early life.

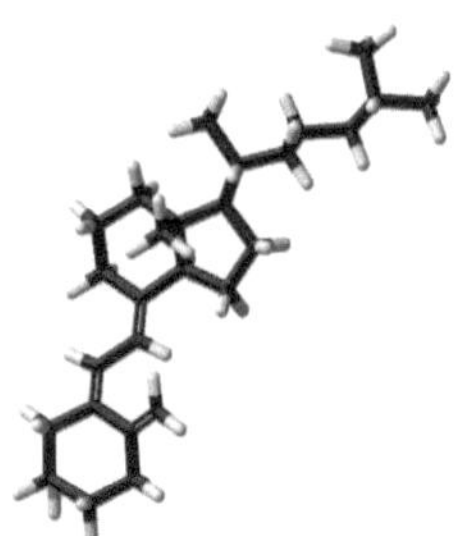

Vitamin D [i2]

Vitamin D also plays an important role in rheumatoid arthritis. Studies show that low vitamin D levels correlate with increased disease activity [s46]. Affected individuals should therefore regularly check their vitamin D status and, if necessary, supplement under medical supervision. The immunmodulatorischen properties of vitamin D are of particular interest [s42]. The vitamin can inhibit the development of autoimmunity and influence the expression of certain receptors [s43]. For example, significant negative correlations between vitamin D levels and <u>autoantibodies</u> have been found in autistic children [s47]. For pregnant women, vitamin D supply is particularly important, as adequate intake during pregnancy can reduce the risk of asthma and other allergic diseases in the child [s45]. Expectant mothers should therefore closely monitor their vitamin D status during pregnancy. The therapeutic possibilities through vitamin D supplementation are promising, although the study situation is still somewhat inconsistent [s48]. An individualized approach, taking into account personal risk profiles and specific autoimmune diseases, is essential.

Practical recommendations for affected individuals:
- Regular monitoring of vitamin D levels, especially with a diagnosed autoimmune disease
- Documentation of disease activity in relation to vitamin D status
- Adjustment of lifestyle habits with sufficient sun exposure
- Balanced diet with vitamin D-rich foods
- Targeted supplementation under medical supervision if necessary

Maintaining adequate vitamin D levels should be understood as a preventive measure against autoimmune diseases [s49]. It should be noted that genetic variation of the vitamin D receptor can influence individual susceptibility to certain diseases [s45].

Autoantibodies

Antibodies that are mistakenly produced by the immune system against the body's own structures and can lead to tissue damage.

Cohort Study

A form of scientific long-term observation in which a specific group of people is studied over an extended period to explore certain developments or correlations.

1. 2. 4. Impact on Mental Health

he impact of vitamin D on mental health is an increasingly important area of research that has received heightened attention in recent years. Scientific studies show a clear correlation between vitamin D deficiency and various mental disorders, particularly depression and anxiety [s50]. Notably, there is a high praevalenz of mental health issues among individuals with vitamin D deficiency. A study of university students found that over 60% of those with a vitamin D deficiency suffered from depression, and about 66% experienced anxiety [s50]. These figures were significantly higher than in the control group with normal vitamin D levels. The biological basis for this connection lies in the important role that vitamin D plays in the brain. The vitamin can cross the bluthirnschranke and is present in brain regions associated with the onset of depression [s51] [s52]. Particularly interesting is vitamin D's ability to regulate neurotrophic factors, which are essential for the survival and function of neurons [s52]. A particularly clear correlation has been demonstrated in young men: An increase in vitamin D concentration by just 10 nmol/L led to an 8% reduction in depression scores [s53]. This underscores the importance of adequate vitamin D supply, especially in young years. A practical tip for students and young professionals would be to take regular breaks outdoors, ideally combined with light physical activity. The connection is especially relevant for individuals with chronic illnesses. For example, in diabetics, it has been shown that vitamin D supplementation has positive effects on mental health [s54]. Affected individuals should therefore regularly check their vitamin D status in consultation with their doctor. Interestingly, a link has also been observed between vitamin D deficiency and the intensity of chronic pain, which in turn affects mental health [s55]. People with chronic pain conditions often report increased depressive symptoms at low vitamin D levels.

The <u>antioxidant</u> properties of vitamin D also play an important role in brain health [s52]. For individuals at increased risk for mental disorders, a preventive vitamin D assessment could be beneficial. A practical approach would be to integrate "vitamin D routines" into daily life, such as:
- Regular walks during lunchtime
- Workplace design near windows
- Conscious planning of outdoor activities
- Balanced diet with vitamin D-rich foods

For clinical practice, this means that vitamin D screening should be considered in the diagnosis and treatment planning of mood disorders [s52]. While the evidence regarding the therapeutic efficacy of vitamin D supplementation for existing mental disorders is still inconclusive, the available data supports a preventive approach. For those affected, it is important to understand that treating a vitamin D deficiency alone does not cure a mental disorder, but it can be a supportive measure within a holistic treatment concept. Supplementation should always be done in consultation with the treating physician and regularly monitored.

Glossary

Antioxidant
Property of a substance that neutralizes harmful free radicals in the body, thereby preventing cell damage

Neurotrophic Factor
Proteins that promote the growth and survival of nerve cells and play an important role in the development of the nervous system

Summary - 1. 2. Vitamin D Deficiency and its Consequences

- Over one billion people worldwide are affected by vitamin D deficiency, with a prevalence of about 40% in Europe.
- In dialysis patients, the prevalence of vitamin D deficiency ranges from 85-99%.
- People with darker skin require longer sun exposure for the same vitamin D production.
- Obesity is a significant risk factor, as body fat binds vitamin D and prevents its absorption into the bloodstream.
- Cholesterol-lowering medications, antiepileptics, and steroids can negatively affect vitamin D metabolism.
- The majority of affected individuals initially show no obvious symptoms.
- A Finnish cohort study showed that children with regular vitamin D supplementation developed type 1 diabetes 80% less frequently.
- In autistic children, significant negative correlations were found between vitamin D levels and autoantibodies.
- Estrogen enhances the effect of vitamin D and leads to a stronger anti-inflammatory response.
- In young men, an increase in vitamin D concentration by 10 nmol/L resulted in an 8% reduction in depression scores.
- 60% of university students with vitamin D deficiency suffered from depression, and 66% from anxiety disorders.
- Vitamin D can cross the blood-brain barrier and regulates neurotrophic factors essential for the survival of neurons.

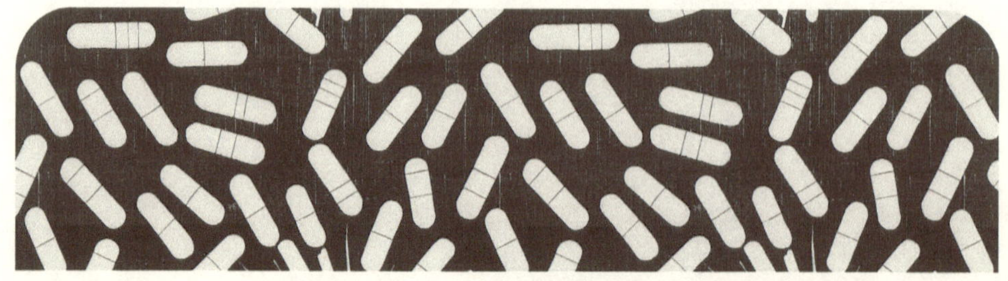

1. 3. Sources of Vitamin D3

he supply of vitamin D3 is a complex interplay of various sources. While our body primarily produces this important vitamin through sunlight, the question arises as to what other options exist to meet our needs. How effective are natural foods as a source of vitamin D? What role do fortified products play in supplementation? And what differences exist between various forms of supplementation? The choice of the right vitamin D source depends on individual factors such as lifestyle, dietary habits, and health conditions. A well-informed understanding of the different sources allows for optimal personal vitamin D supply.

„Fatty fish such as salmon, mackerel, herring, and sardines are the most significant natural source of vitamin D."

1. 3. 1. Natural Sunlight Exposure

atural sunlight exposure is the most important way for the human body to produce Vitamin D3. This process begins when UVB rays from the sun hit our skin and react with the existing 7-dehydrocholesterol [s56]. Initially, pre-vitamin D3 is formed, which subsequently converts into Vitamin D3 and enters the bloodstream over several days [s57]. The efficiency of this endogenous Vitamin D3 production is influenced by numerous factors. Particularly relevant are the latitude of the location, the season, the time of day, and individual factors such as age and skin pigmentation [s58]. For instance, individuals with darker skin may require up to ten times longer to produce the same amount of Vitamin D3 as those with lighter skin [s56]. This should be taken into account when planning individual sunlight exposure. In temperate regions, endogenous Vitamin D3 production is especially seasonal. From late March to late September, most people can meet their entire Vitamin D needs through sunlight [s59]. In the winter months from October to early March, however, UVB radiation is usually too weak for sufficient production [s59]. During this time, supplementary Vitamin D intake through diet or supplements is recommended. For optimal Vitamin D3 production, one should preferably be outdoors between 10 AM and 3 PM [s58]. A sensible sun exposure of 5-30 minutes twice a week, with arms and legs uncovered, may already suffice to meet basic needs [s56]. A practical tip is to use the lunch break for a short walk, exposing the forearms and face to the sun. Interestingly, the Vitamin D produced by sunlight remains active in the body longer than that obtained from supplements [s60]. The body has effective control mechanisms to ensure that only the necessary amount of Vitamin D is produced [s57]. A slight reddening of the skin within 24 hours after sun exposure can already stimulate the production of 15,000-20,000 IU of Vitamin D [s57]. However, skin protection should not be neglected during sun exposure. While sunscreens reduce UVB absorption and thus Vitamin D synthesis [s56], studies show that daily application does not necessarily lead to Vitamin D deficiency [s61]. Even with sunscreen, enough UV rays reach the skin to ensure some Vitamin D production. For individuals who can spend little time outdoors or have specific risk factors, the use of specialized UVB LED technologies may represent an alternative. These emit UVB light with a specific wavelength that is about 3.5 times more effective for Vitamin D production than for causing sunburn [s60].

Such systems can personalize the UVB dose based on individual factors such as skin type and local sunlight availability. Notably, about 77% of the global population has low Vitamin D levels [s57]. This underscores the importance of conscious and regular sunlight exposure as part of a healthy lifestyle. A practical approach is to move daily activities such as phone calls or short meetings outdoors whenever possible to support natural Vitamin D production.

Glossary

UVB Rays

Ultraviolet rays of type B with a wavelength between 280 and 315 nanometers, which make up about 5% of the UV radiation reaching the Earth's surface

1. 3. 2. Vitamin D-rich Foods

he intake of vitamin D through diet plays an important role in overall supply, especially during the sun-poor winter months. However, the number of natural foods that contain significant amounts of vitamin D is limited [s62]. Fatty fish represent the most important natural source, with salmon, mackerel, herring, and sardines being particularly noteworthy [s62] [s63]. To optimize vitamin D intake through fish, it is advisable to include a portion of fatty fish in the diet at least twice a week. A practical tip is to prepare homemade fish spreads, such as from mackerel or

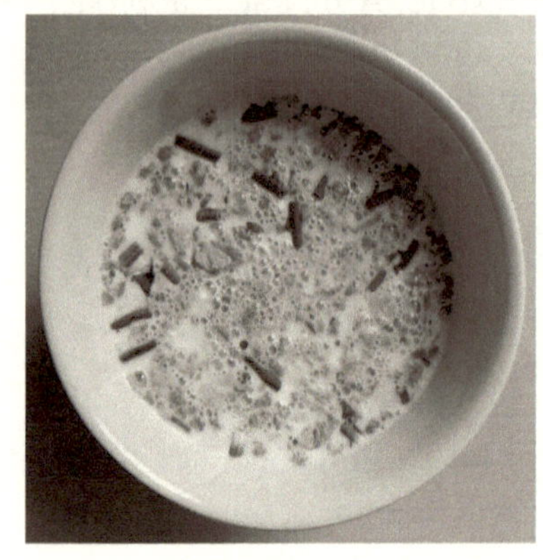

Muesli [i4]

sardines, which make excellent toppings for bread and simultaneously serve as a good source of vitamin D. Egg yolk also contributes to vitamin D supply [s62]. However, one would have to consume unrealistically large amounts of eggs to meet the daily requirement solely through them. Nevertheless, eggs can contribute to overall supply as part of a balanced diet. A creative breakfast with poached eggs on whole grain bread or a homemade scrambled egg with fresh herbs are tasty ways to incorporate vitamin D through egg yolk. Liver also contains vitamin D [s62], although pregnant women should avoid consumption due to the high vitamin A content, which could harm the unborn child. For everyone else, liver can occasionally serve as a source of vitamin D, for example, in traditional dishes like liver sausage or fried liver with onions. Since natural foods alone are often insufficient to meet vitamin D needs, fortified products play an important role. This is particularly evident with milk: natural milk is not a good source of vitamin D [s64], which is why fortification is carried out in many countries. Certain fat spreads and breakfast cereals are also fortified with vitamin D [s62] [s63]. A practical approach for everyday life is the conscious combination of various vitamin D sources. For example, a vitamin D-optimized breakfast could consist of fortified muesli with fortified milk, complemented by an egg and a vitamin D-fortified spread.

For lunch, a fish dish, such as grilled salmon with vegetables, is recommended. When shopping, it is worthwhile to specifically look for fortified products and compare nutritional information. It should be noted that the bioavailability of vitamin D can be improved by simultaneously consuming healthy fats. A trick is to combine vitamin D-rich foods with high-quality oils [s65]. Preparation also plays an important role: vitamin D is relatively heat-stable; however, vitamin D-rich foods should be prepared gently. For fish, steaming or briefly frying over medium heat is recommended to best preserve the valuable nutrients. For people who follow a vegetarian or vegan diet, obtaining sufficient vitamin D through food is particularly challenging, as the richest natural sources are of animal origin. Here, fortified products and alternative strategies, such as vitamin D-fortified plant drinks, gain special importance.

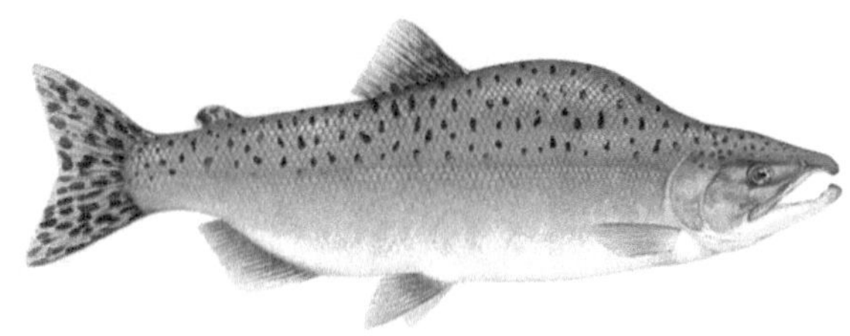

Salmon [i3]

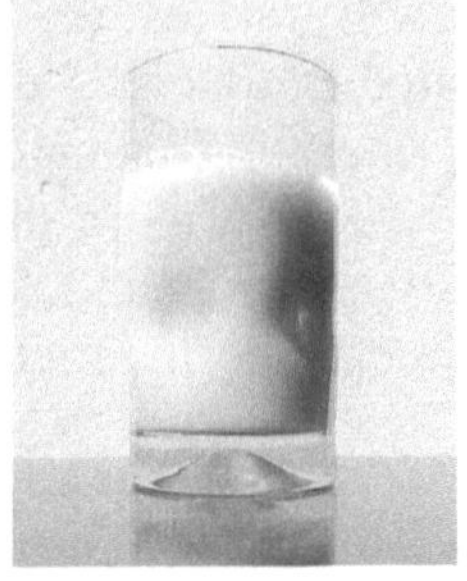

Plant-based drink [i5]

1. 3. 3. Fortified Foods

The systematic fortification of foods with vitamin D has a long history, dating back to the 1930s. This measure was first introduced to combat the widespread occurrence of rickets [s66]. Since then, food fortification has established itself as an important strategy for improving the vitamin D supply in the population. The effectiveness of this measure has been demonstrated in various studies. For instance, one investigation showed that individuals who regularly consumed vitamin D3-fortified foods were able to maintain stable vitamin D levels even during the winter months, while a seasonal decline was observed in the control group [s67]. This underscores the significant role of fortified foods, especially during times of low sunlight. Interestingly, there are notable international differences in fortification practices. For example, in the United Kingdom, cow's milk is not routinely fortified with vitamin D [s68], whereas this is common practice in other countries. Therefore, it is important for consumers to know that the vitamin D content of similar products can vary significantly depending on the country of origin. A practical tip is to pay attention to the nutritional information when shopping, as fortification with vitamin D must be clearly indicated [s69]. Fortification primarily occurs in two forms: as vitamin D2 or D3 [s66]. Both forms are effective, although vitamin D3 is somewhat better utilized by the body. When selecting fortified products, consumers should keep the recommended daily doses in mind, which are 5 μg (200 IU) for adults and 10 μg (400 IU) during growth phases [s70]. A particularly interesting example of traditionally fortified products is cod liver oil [s71], which has been used for generations for vitamin D supplementation. However, modern fortification strategies are significantly more diverse and encompass a wide range of foods. To optimize vitamin D intake, it is advisable to cleverly integrate various fortified products into the diet.

Practical tips for everyday life:
- Combine fortified cereals with fortified plant milk for breakfast
- Use fortified margarine or spreads
- Pay attention to processed foods labeled "fortified with vitamin D"
- Keep a food diary to track the consumption of fortified products
- Educate yourself about local fortification practices, especially during stays abroad

The systematic fortification of foods is continuously evaluated and adjusted by expert groups [s67]. This ensures that fortification programs remain effective and safe. For consumers, this means they can trust fortified foods as part of a balanced diet. Another important aspect is the combination of various vitamin D sources. Fortified foods should not be considered the sole source but rather a meaningful supplement to natural vitamin D sources and sunlight exposure. This is particularly relevant for individuals with increased vitamin D needs or limited access to natural sources. The development of new fortification technologies and strategies is continuously progressing, leading to an ever-growing selection of fortified products. This provides consumers with more opportunities to optimize and tailor their vitamin D supply.

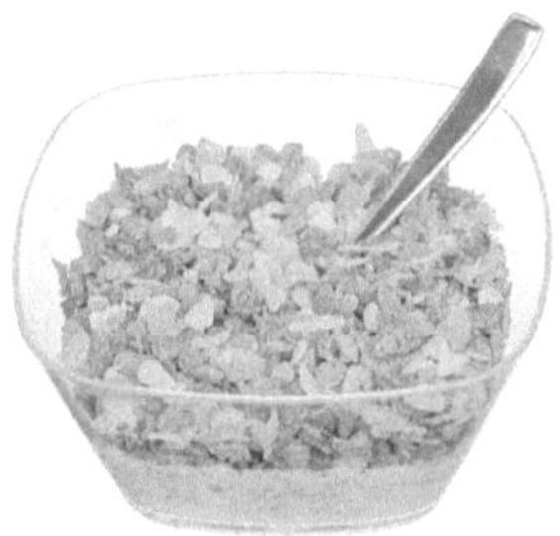

Cereals [i6]

1. 3. 4. Various Forms of Vitamin D3 Supplements

itamin D3 supplements are available in various forms that differ in their application and bioavailability. The most common forms are tablets, capsules, and drops [s72]. This variety allows for individual adaptation of supplementation to personal needs and preferences. Liquid preparations in the form of drops offer several advantages. They are particularly suitable for individuals with swallowing difficulties or for young children. Additionally, they can be dosed very precisely, which is especially important for infants who require 400 IU of vitamin D daily [s73]. A practical tip for parents is to administer the vitamin D drops directly onto the pacifier or mix them with some expressed breast milk. Tablets and capsules are the classic forms of administration and are particularly suitable for adults. They are easy to handle and allow for standardized dosing. For individuals with swallowing difficulties, chewable tablets or dissolvable variants are also available. It should be noted that vitamin D is fat-soluble; therefore, absorption is improved when the supplements are taken with a fatty meal. Vitamin D supplements are particularly important for individuals with fat absorption disorders, lactose intolerance, or milk allergies [s74]. For these groups, special formulations are available that ensure better absorption. A practical approach here is the use of microencapsulated preparations or oil-based drops. The dosage of the supplements should be tailored to individual needs. While the general recommendation for adults is 15 mcg (600 IU), older individuals over 70 years require 20 mcg (800 IU) daily [s73]. In cases of proven deficiency or specific risk factors, higher doses may also be necessary [s75]. An important biochemical aspect is the conversion of the ingested vitamin in the body. Both vitamin D3 and D2 are initially converted into 25-hydroxyvitamin D (calcidiol) before activation to $1\alpha,25$-dihydroxyvitamin D (calcitriol) occurs in the kidneys [s76]. These metabolic pathways should be considered when choosing a supplement.

For practical application, a systematic approach is recommended:
- Choose a form of administration that fits your lifestyle
- Take the supplement regularly at the same time each day
- Document the intake in a calendar or an app
- Have your vitamin D levels checked regularly
- Store the supplements in a cool, light-protected place

The choice of the right supplement should be made in consultation with medical professionals, especially if there are existing health limitations. Possible interactions with other medications should also be considered.

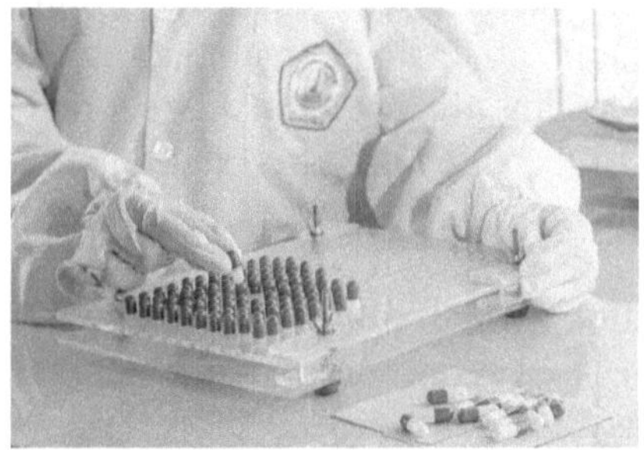

Capsules [i7]

1. 3. 5. Differences between Vitamin D2 and D3

he two most important forms of vitamin D - vitamin D2 (Ergocalciferol) and vitamin D3 (Cholecalciferol) - differ significantly in their origin and effectiveness [s77]. While vitamin D2 is primarily produced by plants, fungi, and <u>invertebrates</u>, vitamin D3 is the form that the human body can produce itself [s78]. A key difference lies in the chemical structure: vitamin D3 has an additional double bond and a <u>methyl group</u>, which explains its higher effectiveness [s78]. These structural differences result in approximately 87% better efficacy of vitamin D3 in raising and maintaining vitamin D levels in the blood. Practically, this means that vitamin D3 supplements allow for 2 to 3 times higher storage in the body compared to equivalent amounts of vitamin D2 [s79]. The different binding affinity to the vitamin D-binding protein is another important aspect. Vitamin D3 binds more strongly to this transport protein, leading to better availability in the body [s78]. A practical tip for consumers is therefore to prefer vitamin D3 supplements when choosing dietary supplements, as these are utilized more efficiently by the body. The degradation rate also plays a significant role: vitamin D2 is broken down faster than vitamin D3, allowing the latter to remain in the body longer and exert its effects [s78]. For individuals looking to optimize their vitamin D intake, this means that they can achieve longer dosing intervals with vitamin D3 supplements. Interestingly for vegetarians and vegans, vitamin D2 is found in some plants and particularly in mushrooms that have been exposed to UVB radiation [s80] [s77]. However, they should be aware of its lower efficacy and may need to consider higher doses or look for vegan vitamin D3 supplements derived from lichens. In blood tests, the amounts of vitamin D2 and D3 can be measured separately [s81], which is important for individual dose adjustment. This allows for precise monitoring of vitamin D status and aids in optimizing supplementation. Most scientific studies confirm the superior efficacy of vitamin D3 over D2 in raising blood vitamin D levels, although some studies have found no significant differences [s78]. For practical application, it is still advisable to prefer vitamin D3 whenever possible. A practical approach for everyday life is the combination of various vitamin D sources: while one primarily absorbs vitamin D3 through sunlight and animal products, one can also obtain vitamin D2 by consuming mushrooms. However, when supplementing, one should primarily focus on vitamin D3 supplements to benefit from the better efficacy. For individuals with specific health conditions or increased vitamin D needs, choosing the right form of vitamin D is particularly important. In such cases, supplementation should be coordinated with a health expert who can also consider individual needs and possible contraindications.

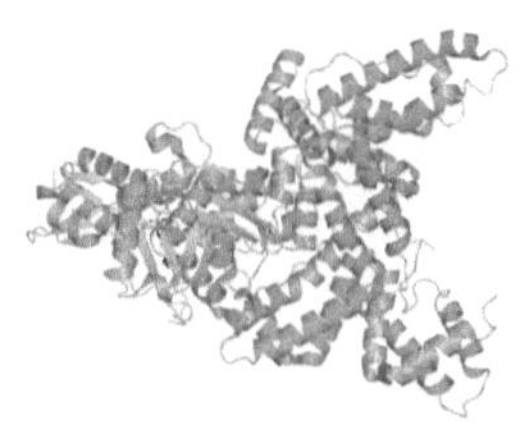

Vitamin D-binding protein [i8]

Glossary

Cholecalciferol
The natural form of vitamin D that is formed in the skin from 7-dehydrocholesterol.

Ergocalciferol
A fat-soluble vitamin that is produced from ergosterol through UV irradiation and is primarily found in fungi.

Invertebrate
Invertebrate animals such as insects, worms, or mollusks that do not possess an internal skeleton.

Methyl group
A chemical group consisting of one carbon atom and three hydrogen atoms, important for many biological processes.

Summary - 1. 3. Sources of Vitamin D3

- UVB rays react with 7-dehydrocholesterol in the skin to form pre-vitamin D3.
- People with dark skin require up to ten times longer for the same vitamin D3 production.
- A slight reddening of the skin can stimulate the production of 15,000-20,000 IU of vitamin D.
- 77% of the global population has low vitamin D levels.
- UVB LED technologies are 3.5 times more effective in vitamin D production than in causing sunburn.
- The bioavailability of vitamin D is improved by the simultaneous intake of healthy fats.
- The systematic fortification of foods with vitamin D began in the 1930s.
- Vitamin D3 allows for 2 to 3 times higher storage in the body than vitamin D2.
- Vitamin D2 is primarily produced by plants, fungi, and invertebrates.
- The additional double bond and methyl group in vitamin D3 explain its 87% higher efficacy.
- Vitamin D3 binds more strongly to the vitamin D-binding transport protein.
- Vitamin D2 is broken down more quickly than vitamin D3.
- Vegan vitamin D3 can be derived from lichens.

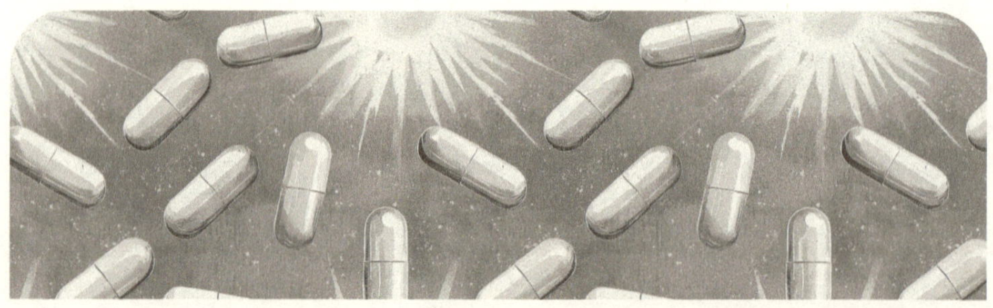

Review - 1. Basics of Vitamin D3 Supplementation

- The formation of vitamin D3 in the skin occurs through UVB radiation from 7-dehydrocholesterol, with efficiency strongly depending on skin type and geographical location.

- Individuals with skin type VI require about five times longer than those with skin type I to produce the same amount of vitamin D.

- The activation of vitamin D3 occurs in a two-step process in the liver and kidneys, regulated by various hormones such as parathyroid hormone and FGF23.

- Without vitamin D, only 10-15% of dietary calcium can be absorbed; with sufficient vitamin D, the absorption rate increases to 30-40%.

- Vitamin D3 regulates approximately 900 different genes and has extensive effects on the immune system, muscle strength, and mental health.

- In diabetics, vitamin D3 supplementation has shown positive effects on mental health.

- The efficiency of the body's own vitamin D production decreases with age, as the skin contains less 7-DHC.

- Vitamin D3 is about 87% more effective than D2 in raising blood levels and is better stored in the body.

- High-dose vitamin D3 supplementation led to a 34% increase in serum levels and a 13% improvement in muscle strength within just 8 days in studies.

- Activated immune cells can locally activate vitamin D, supporting their defense function.

- Optimal supply of this essential vitamin depends on the correct dosage—more on this in the next chapter on the practical application of vitamin D3.

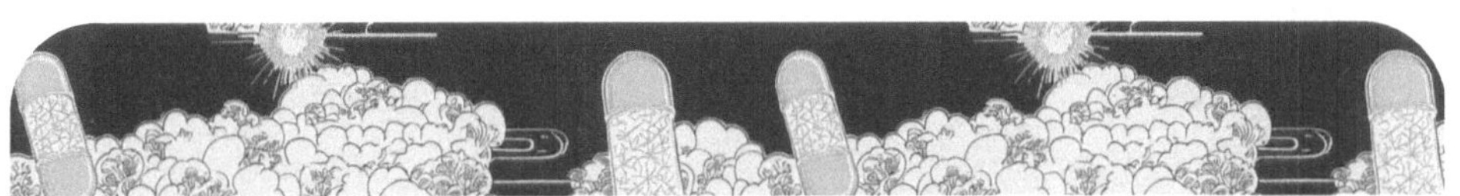

2. Dosage and Application of Vitamin D3

he correct dosage and application of Vitamin D3 raises questions for many people: When is the best time to take it? Which form of administration is most suitable? And how much Vitamin D3 do different groups of people actually need? The answers to these questions are complex, as optimal Vitamin D3 supply depends on numerous individual factors. Age, weight, skin type, and pre-existing conditions all play a role, as do the geographical location of one's residence and personal lifestyle habits. The season also significantly influences the need. Particularly relevant is the question of potential risks: When does sensible supplementation become a potentially dangerous overdose? What interactions can occur with other medications? And how can Vitamin D levels be reliably monitored? Recent scientific findings have significantly expanded our understanding of optimal Vitamin D3 supply. What was once considered sufficient is often regarded today as too low. These new insights allow for a more precise and individualized dosage—provided one is aware of the crucial factors.

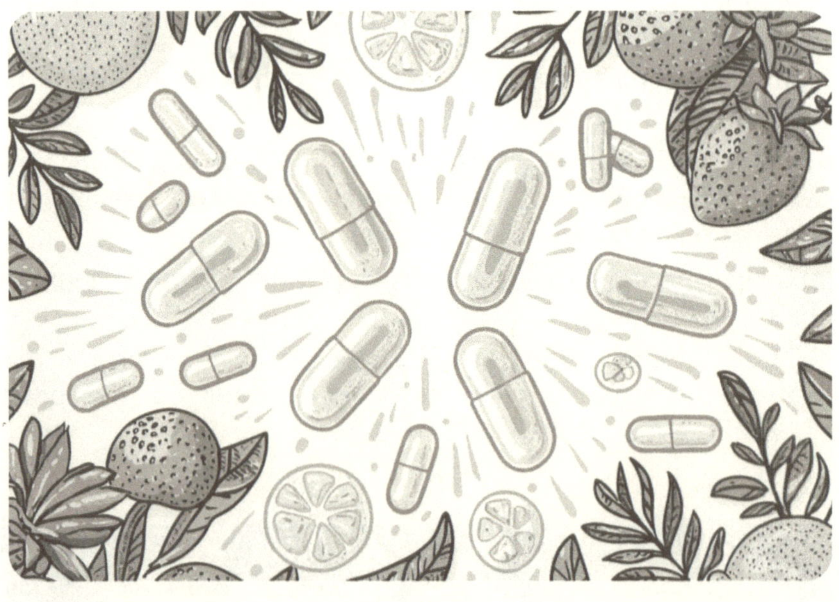

2. 1. Recommended Daily Dose

he question of the correct dosage of vitamin D3 has occupied physicians and scientists for years. How much does the body actually need? Why do the recommendations of different health organizations sometimes differ significantly? And why is the natural production of vitamin D through sunlight insufficient for many people? The answers to these questions are complex and depend on numerous individual factors. Age, weight, skin type, lifestyle, and any pre-existing conditions play an important role in determining personal vitamin D3 needs. While standardized recommendations may suffice for some individuals, others require significantly higher doses. Current scientific findings on optimal vitamin D3 supply open new perspectives for individualized supplementation that goes far beyond the classical standard recommendations.

„*The safe upper intake limit for adults is 4000 IU (100 micrograms) per day.*"

2. 1. 1. General Recommendations for Adults

he recommendations for daily vitamin D3 intake in adults vary depending on age, life situation, and various health factors. For healthy adults aged 19 to 70 years, a daily dose of 600 IE (International Units) or 15 micrograms is generally recommended [s82]. From the age of 71, this recommendation increases to 800 IE (20 micrograms) daily, as older individuals may absorb and metabolize vitamin D and calcium less efficiently [s83]. However, recent research suggests that these standard recommendations may be set too low. Some experts recommend a higher daily intake between 1500 and 2000 IE to maintain an optimal 25-hydroxyvitamin D level of at least 30 ng/mL in the blood [s84]. This is particularly relevant for individuals who spend little time outdoors or live in regions with low sunlight. In such cases, the daily intake should be at least 1000 IE [s85]. For practical implementation, this means that individuals who work in an office and primarily stay indoors should pay particular attention to adequate vitamin D supply, especially during the autumn and winter months. A daily 15-minute walk at midday with uncovered hands and face can already be helpful. Nevertheless, in many cases, additional supplementation is advisable. The safe upper intake limit for adults is 4000 IE (100 micrograms) per day [s82]. Interestingly, studies show that even a daily intake of up to 5000 IE does not cause serious side effects [s86]. However, supplementation above 2000 IE should only be done after consulting medical professionals. For pregnant and breastfeeding women, the same basic recommendations apply as for other adults: 600 IE daily [s87]. However, they should monitor their vitamin D supply particularly carefully, as the demand may be increased during these life stages. An important aspect is the monitoring of vitamin D levels in the blood. A value of at least 50 nmol/L (20 ng/mL) is considered sufficient for bone health [s82]. However, optimal values are 70 nmol/L or higher, as these are associated with various health benefits [s88]. To achieve these values, it may be sensible to determine one's vitamin D status through a blood test and adjust supplementation accordingly. Practical tips for everyday life: In addition to supplementation, vitamin D supply can be supported by regular outdoor exercise. It should be noted that sunscreen can reduce the body's own vitamin D production. A balanced diet with vitamin D-rich foods such as fatty fish, eggs, and fortified dairy products can also contribute to overall supply, although diet alone is usually not sufficient to meet the full requirement. Particularly individuals with darker skin, those who are overweight, or people who cover their skin for cultural or health reasons should pay special attention to their vitamin D supply and consider higher dosages if necessary [s89].

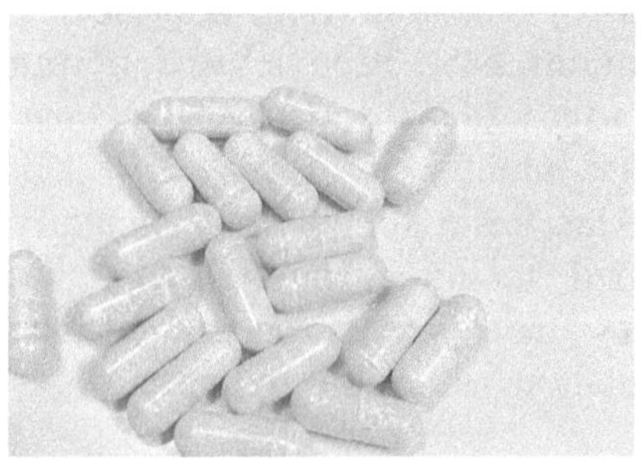

Supplementation [i9]

Glossary

International Unit
A standardized unit of measurement for biologically active substances, internationally established to uniformly measure the potency of vitamins and other substances.

Nanogram per Milliliter
A concentration measurement that corresponds to one billionth of a gram per milliliter and is often used when measuring very small amounts of substances.

Nanomole per Liter
A unit of concentration in the international system of units, indicating the amount of substance in nanomoles per liter.

2. 1. 2. Dosage for Children and Adolescents

itamin D3 supply plays an important role in the healthy development of children and adolescents from birth. Current recommendations have been revised upwards in recent years, as previous dosages of 200 IU were deemed too low [s90]. For newborns in their first month of life, a daily dose of 300-400 IU is recommended [s91]. This basic supply is particularly important, as infants should not be exposed to direct sunlight in the first weeks of life. Practically, this means that parents should ideally discuss and initiate vitamin D3 supplementation with their pediatrician immediately after birth.

From the second month of life until the age of 18, the recommended daily dose ranges from 400 to 1,000 IU [s91]. The following age-specific guidelines apply:
- Infants 0-6 months: 400 IU (10 μg) daily
- Infants 7-12 months: 400 IU (10 μg) daily
- Toddlers 1-3 years: 600 IU (15 μg) daily
- Children 4-8 years: 600 IU (15 μg) daily [s92]

Supplementation is particularly important for children who consume less than one liter of vitamin D-fortified milk per day [s93]. In practice, this affects most children, as such high milk consumption is rather unusual. Therefore, parents should pay special attention to adequate vitamin D3 supply, especially during the winter months.

In cases of proven vitamin D deficiency, significantly higher dosages may be required. Therapeutic doses vary by age group:
- Up to 1 year: 1,000-3,000 IU daily
- 1-12 years: 3,000-6,000 IU daily
- 12-18 years: 6,000-10,000 IU daily [s91]

Such high dosages should only be administered under medical supervision and after regular monitoring of blood values. To avoid overdoses, the following upper limits (<u>UL</u> - Upper Level) have been established:
- Infants 0-6 months: 1,000 IU (25 μg)
- Infants 7-12 months: 1,500 IU (38 μg)
- Toddlers 1-3 years: 2,500 IU (63 μg)
- Children 4-8 years: 3,000 IU (75 μg) [s92]

For practical implementation in daily life, it is advisable to establish fixed routines. The administration of vitamin D3 can, for example, be associated with the morning breakfast or the evening tooth brushing. For infants, it is suitable to administer it during one of the meals. Supplementation should occur year-round, even if children spend a lot of time outdoors.

Parents should pay special attention to vitamin D supply in:
- Children with dark skin
- Children who predominantly stay indoors
- Children who wear covering clothing for cultural or health reasons
- Children with limited sun exposure
- Overweight children

Supplementation should be complemented by regular outdoor activity. A good compromise between sun protection and vitamin D production is to allow children to play outside for about 10-15 minutes with uncovered forearms and legs during the morning or later afternoon hours. However, sunburn should be strictly avoided. Regular monitoring of vitamin D status by the pediatrician is advisable, especially for at-risk groups or when signs of deficiency are present. This allows for individual adjustment of the dosage as needed to ensure optimal supply.

Glossary

Upper Level

Refers to the maximum safe daily intake of a nutrient, at which no health risks are expected. Established by health authorities.

2. 1. 3. Dose Adjustment for Seniors

eniors have an increased need for vitamin D3, as their skin becomes less efficient at producing vitamin D with age, and intestinal absorption declines [s94]. Therefore, adjusting the dosage for this age group is particularly important to minimize health risks and maintain quality of life. Current research shows that a daily intake of 800 to 1000 IU of vitamin D3 significantly reduces the fall risk in older adults by 22% [s95]. Even more impressive are the results with a dosage of 700 to 1000 IU daily, which can lower the fall risk by 34% [s96]. These findings are especially relevant for seniors living in care facilities or those with a history of falls. For optimal supplementation, experts recommend a daily dose of 2000 IU (50 µg) for individuals over 70 years old [s94]. This higher dosage accounts for the age-related decline in the body's vitamin D production. In practical terms, this means that seniors can ideally distribute their vitamin D3 supplementation into two doses per day—one in the morning and one in the evening, each taken with meals. Interestingly, studies show that an even higher daily dose of 4000 IU led to an optimal blood level of over 90 nmol/L in 88% of participants after one year, while this was only the case for 70% at 2000 IU [s97]. However, such high dosages should only be taken after consulting with a healthcare provider and under regular monitoring of blood levels. Regularity of intake is particularly important. Studies have shown that intermittent dosing, such as taking a higher dose once a month, has no preventive effect on falls [s95]. A practical tip is to use a medication dispenser with weekly divisions, which facilitates daily intake and helps establish a routine. For seniors with osteoporosis, vitamin D3 supplementation is especially critical. The minimum dose should not fall below 700-800 IU per day [s98]. In combination with calcium, this dosage has proven effective in reducing the risk of <u>fragility fractures</u> [s99]. A practical approach is to take it during breakfast along with calcium-rich foods like dairy products.

Most older adults tolerate a daily dose of 800 IU very well and have a low risk of side effects [s100]. Nevertheless, certain factors should be considered in individual dosing:
- Skin type and sun exposure
- Degree of mobility and time spent outdoors
- Dietary habits
- Comorbidities
- Medication use

For practical implementation in daily life, the following approach is recommended: 1. Determine vitamin D status through a blood test 2. Discuss individual dosing with a physician 3. Establish a daily intake routine 4. Engage in regular outdoor activity, ideally in the morning 5. Maintain a balanced diet with vitamin D-rich foods 6. Regularly monitor blood levels, especially at the beginning of the supplementation

Seniors should pay special attention to their vitamin D3 intake if they:
- Primarily live indoors
- Have mobility limitations
- Take multiple medications
- Suffer from chronic illnesses
- Have impaired kidney function

Supplementation should be understood as part of a holistic health concept that also includes regular exercise, a balanced diet, and social activities.

Fragility Fracture

A bone fracture that occurs even with minimal stress or a slight fall, typically due to reduced bone density. Most commonly occurs in the wrist, hip, and spine.

Supplementation

The additional intake of nutrients in the form of supplements to complement the normal diet. Can occur in various forms such as tablets, capsules, or drops.

2. 1. 4. Special Needs During Pregnancy

uring pregnancy, adequate vitamin D3 supply is of particular importance, as it influences not only the health of the expectant mother but also the optimal development of the unborn child. Current research findings indicate that a vitamin D deficiency during pregnancy can be associated with significant health risks [s101]. For optimal supply, pregnant women are recommended to supplement with 10 micrograms (400 IU) of vitamin D3 daily [s102]. However, recent studies suggest that higher doses between 1000 and 4000 IU daily may be more beneficial for achieving better health outcomes for both mother and child [s103]. An optimal vitamin D level in the blood (25-OH-D) should be at least 100 nmoll (40 ngml) [s104]. Notably, the preventive effect of adequate vitamin D supply is remarkable: supplementation can significantly reduce the risk of pregnancy-related complications. Specifically, it has been demonstrated that the risk of preeclampsia can be reduced by 60%, the risk of gestational diabetes by 50%, and the risk of preterm birth by 40% [s101]. These findings underscore the importance of consistent supplementation. For practical implementation in daily life, the following approach is recommended: 1. Supplementation with vitamin D3 should begin as soon as pregnancy is confirmed. Ideally, the intake should occur at the same time each day, for example, at breakfast, to establish it as a routine. 2. Supplementation should occur year-round, with particular attention to consistent intake during the autumn and winter months (September to March) [s105] [s106]. 3. Many pregnancy multivitamin preparations already contain vitamin D3. These are provided free of charge in many countries for the duration of the pregnancy [s102]. Pregnant women should discuss with their midwife or doctor whether the amount included is sufficient or if additional supplementation would be advisable. 4. In addition to supplementation, a balanced, calcium-rich diet is important, as vitamin D3 regulates the absorption and utilization of calcium in the body [s105]. This is essential for the development of healthy bones, teeth, and muscles in the unborn child. 5. Moderate outdoor exercise should be part of the daily routine, taking appropriate sun protection into account. A 15-20 minute walk in the morning hours can contribute to the body's own vitamin D production.

Pregnant women should pay special attention to their vitamin D supply if they:
- have darker skin
- spend most of their time indoors
- wear covering clothing
- are overweight
- follow a vegan or vegetarian diet

Regular monitoring of vitamin D levels by the attending physician is advisable, especially at the beginning of pregnancy and for risk groups. This allows for individual dosage adjustments as needed to ensure optimal supply. Supplementation should be understood as part of a holistic health concept during pregnancy, which also includes balanced nutrition, moderate exercise, and adequate rest. The positive impact on the health of both mother and child justifies the relatively small effort of daily supplementation.

Glossary

Gestational Diabetes
A form of diabetes that occurs for the first time during pregnancy and is characterized by impaired glucose tolerance. It usually resolves after childbirth.

Preeclampsia
A pregnancy-related condition characterized by high blood pressure and protein in the urine. If untreated, it can become life-threatening for both mother and child.

2. 1. 5. Consideration of Pre-existing Conditions

n certain pre-existing conditions, the Vitamin D3 dosage must be individually adjusted, as these conditions can influence Vitamin D metabolism or cause an increased need. Medical monitoring of Vitamin D levels is particularly important in these cases [s107]. Patients with gastrointestinal diseases such as zoeliakie or inflammatory bowel diseases often have difficulties absorbing Vitamin D. In these conditions, close monitoring of blood values and usually a higher dosage are required [s107]. In practice, this means that affected individuals should ideally combine their supplementation with high-fat meals to improve absorption. In liver diseases such as biliary cirrhosis or liver cirrhosis, the activation of Vitamin D in the body is impaired. These patients require particularly careful monitoring of their Vitamin D levels [s107]. The dosage must be individually adjusted, taking liver function values into account. Patients with diabetes mellitus often have an increased need for Vitamin D [s108]. Optimal supply can contribute to better blood sugar control. Diabetics should therefore pay special attention to regular monitoring of their Vitamin D levels and coordinate supplementation with their diabetes therapy. In obesity, especially after bariatrischer_chirurgie, higher Vitamin D doses are required [s108]. This is because Vitamin D is stored in adipose tissue, making less available for metabolism. Affected individuals should ideally distribute their Vitamin D supplementation over several smaller doses throughout the day. Particular attention should be given to patients treated with glucocorticoids (cortisone). A daily dose of 2000 IU is recommended for them to achieve a 25-hydroxyvitamin D level of at least 32 ng/mL [s108]. The intake should ideally not occur simultaneously with glucocorticoids but rather staggered to optimize absorption. For osteoporosis patients, adequate Vitamin D supply is particularly critical for therapeutic success [s107]. Supplementation should always be combined with calcium and regularly monitored through bone density measurements and Vitamin D level checks. For practical implementation in cases of pre-existing conditions, the following approach is recommended: 1. Regular monitoring of Vitamin D levels, at least every 3-6 months 2. Documentation of intake and any symptoms 3. Coordination of supplementation with other medications 4. Adjustment of dosage according to blood values and disease progression 5. Consideration of interactions with other medications Supplementation in cases of pre-existing conditions should only occur under medical supervision. It is important for patients to inform their treating physician about all medications and dietary supplements taken to avoid potential interactions.

62

glucocorticoid
Endogenous or artificially produced hormones with anti-inflammatory and immunosuppressive effects

Summary - 2. 1. Recommended Daily Dose

- The recommended daily dose for adults aged 19-70 years is 600 IU, which increases to 800 IU from the age of 71.
- Recent research recommends 1500-2000 IU daily for an optimal 25-hydroxyvitamin D level of at least 30 ng/mL.
- The safe upper intake limit is 4000 IU per day, with studies showing that up to 5000 IU do not cause serious side effects.
- For newborns in the first month of life, 300-400 IU is recommended, and thereafter until the age of 18, 400-1000 IU.
- In cases of proven vitamin D deficiency, therapeutic doses of 6000-10000 IU may be necessary for those aged 12-18.
- A daily intake of 800-1000 IU reduces the risk of falls in older adults by 22%, and by 34% at 700-1000 IU.
- 4000 IU daily resulted in an optimal blood level above 90 nmol/L in 88% of study participants after one year.
- During pregnancy, adequate vitamin D supply can reduce the risk of preeclampsia by 60% and the risk of gestational diabetes by 50%.
- In cases of obesity and after bariatric surgery, higher vitamin D doses are necessary, as the vitamin is stored in adipose tissue.
- Patients undergoing glucocorticoid therapy require 2000 IU daily for a 25-hydroxyvitamin D level of at least 32 ng/mL.

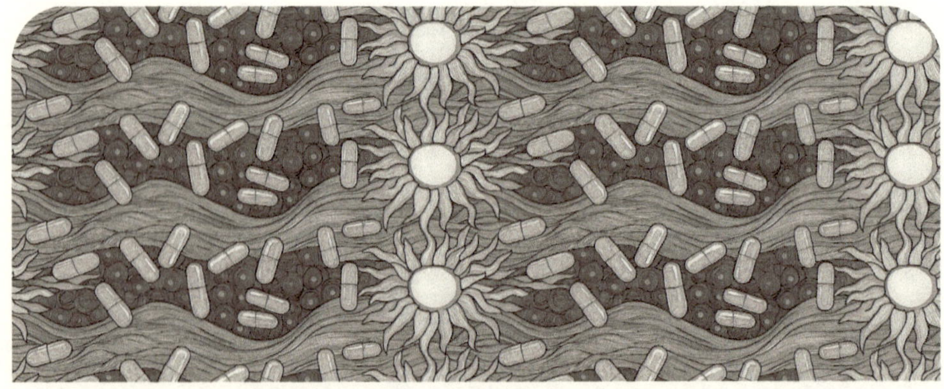

2. 2. High-dose Vitamin D3 Supplementation

he high-dose supplementation of Vitamin D3 raises numerous questions: When is it medically advisable? What risks does it entail? How can the optimal dosage for the individual patient be determined? Recent scientific research has shown that certain groups of people can benefit from high-dose therapy. At the same time, this form of supplementation requires special attention regarding potential side effects and interactions with other medications. The correct implementation of high-dose Vitamin D3 supplementation is based on precise medical indications, careful monitoring, and individual dosage adjustment. A solid understanding of these aspects is equally important for both therapists and patients to ensure the treatment is safe and effective. The following sections illuminate the various facets of high-dose therapy and provide evidence-based recommendations for practical application.

„With a high-dose vitamin D3 supplementation of 3200-4000 IU daily, the risk of hypercalcemia is 4 cases per 1000 individuals.“

2. 2. 1. Indications for high-dose Vitamin D3

igh-dose Vitamin D3 supplementation is employed as a therapeutic measure for various medical conditions and risk groups. The indications are based on scientific findings and clinical experiences. A primary reason for high-dose therapy is a documented severe Vitamin D deficiency, with 25-hydroxyvitamin D levels below 20 ng/mL [s109]. This is particularly common among certain risk groups. Studies indicate that in the USA, 50% of children aged 1-5 years and even 70% of those aged 6-11 years exhibit Vitamin D deficiency [s110]. In cases of malabsorption syndromes, such as those occurring in chronic inflammatory bowel diseases (Crohn's disease, ulcerative colitis), significantly higher doses of Vitamin D3 are often required [s109] [s111]. A practical example: a patient with Crohn's disease may need three to four times the usual supplementation dose to achieve an adequate Vitamin D level. Particular attention is given to patients following bariatric procedures. Here, a minimum of 3000 IU daily is recommended to reach a target value of 28 ng/mL [s111]. Treating physicians should regularly monitor Vitamin D levels and adjust the dosage accordingly. For cystic fibrosis patients aged 2 years and older with pancreatic insufficiency, high-dose therapy is indicated if adequate levels are not achieved after six months of standard supplementation [s112]. The dosage is determined individually based on age and current 25-OHD levels.

Other important indications include:
- Osteoporosis and increased fracture risk (recommended daily dose: 800-2000 IU) [s113]
- Patients undergoing corticosteroid therapy (target dose: 2000 IU daily) [s111]
- Severe kidney diseases (stages III-V) [s114]
- Liver diseases such as biliary cirrhosis [s114]

Preventive supplementation is recommended for pregnant women, breastfeeding mothers, and older adults [s113]. A Vitamin D deficiency during pregnancy can negatively impact the child's bone development [s110]. Individuals with darker skin tones (African Americans, Hispanics) and those with obesity are also particularly at risk [s110]. In obese patients, especially after weight-reducing surgeries, the dosage must be adjusted accordingly [s111]. Routine testing of Vitamin D levels is not recommended [s113]. However, measurement is indicated in the presence of specific risk factors or symptoms such as unexplained bone pain, unusual fractures, or signs of metabolic bone disorders [s113]. In high-dose therapy, it is important to note that it should be avoided in patients with a 25-OHD level ≥30 ng/mL or a corrected calcium >10.5 mg/dl [s112]. Treatment should always be conducted under medical supervision to prevent overdose. For patients with primary hyperparathyroidism, Vitamin D supplementation is recommended to control PTH levels, aiming for values above 30 ng/mL [s111]. This underscores the importance of regular monitoring of relevant laboratory parameters during high-dose therapy.

Glossary

hyperparathyroidism
Overactivity of the parathyroid glands leading to increased production of parathyroid hormone

2. 2. 2. Risks and Side Effects

igh-dose vitamin D3 supplementation carries various risks and potential side effects that must be carefully considered. The most significant complication is <u>hypercalcemia</u> - an excessive accumulation of calcium in the blood [s115]. This may initially manifest through nonspecific symptoms such as increased thirst, frequent urination (<u>polyuria</u>), loss of appetite, and nausea [s116]. For instance, one patient reported that he initially only experienced increased thirst, mistakenly attributing it to the warm weather - it was only the blood test at the doctor's office that revealed dangerously elevated calcium levels. The risk of overdose is particularly present with independent, uncontrolled supplementation. Scientific data indicate that with high-dose supplementation of 3200-4000 IU daily, the risk of hypercalcemia is 4 cases per 1000 individuals [s117]. This underscores the importance of regular medical monitoring of relevant blood values. Particular caution is warranted in dosing for different age groups. While the safe upper intake limit for adults and children aged 9 and older is 100 micrograms (4000 IU) per day [s118], significantly lower limits apply to younger age groups: children aged 1-10 should receive a maximum of 50 micrograms daily, and infants under 12 months should not exceed 25 micrograms [s115]. A practical example: a 2-year-old child should never receive the same dose as an adult, even in the presence of proven vitamin D deficiency. Long-term consequences of overdose can be severe. Chronic toxicity can lead to kidney damage in the form of <u>nephrocalcinosis</u> [s119]. Paradoxically, bone health may also be compromised, as elevated vitamin D levels can lead to increased calcium mobilization from the bones [s116]. In extreme cases, seizures and disturbances of consciousness, even leading to coma, have been observed [s120]. An often-overlooked aspect is the delayed manifestation of overdose symptoms. These may develop weeks to months after the onset of excessive intake [s116]. This makes early detection particularly challenging and underscores the importance of preventive checks. A warning signal is a 25hydroxyvitamin_d level above 125 nmol/L, which is considered too high [s118]. Individuals taking multiple vitamin D-containing preparations simultaneously are particularly at risk. A typical example is the combination of vitamin D drops with multivitamin supplements or fortified foods. Care should be taken to monitor the total intake amount. The issue is exacerbated by the fact that vitamin D can be stored in the body as a fat-soluble vitamin [s121]. Unlike water-soluble vitamins, an excess is not simply excreted but can accumulate in tissues. This also explains why chronic overdose is particularly dangerous.

Practical recommendations for risk minimization:
- Keep a supplementation diary with all vitamin D sources
- Regularly (every 3-6 months) check your vitamin D and calcium levels
- Pay attention to early warning signs such as increased thirst or fatigue
- Inform all treating physicians about your supplementation
- Avoid simultaneous intake of various vitamin D-containing preparations

Supplementation should always be conducted under medical supervision, as the individually correct dose depends on many factors and overdose must be avoided [s121]. This is especially true for at-risk groups such as pregnant women, children, and the elderly.

Glossary

Hypercalcemia
A metabolic disorder in which the calcium level in the blood is abnormally elevated. Can be caused by vitamin D overdose as well as tumors or hormonal disorders.

Nephrocalcinosis
Abnormal deposition of calcium salts in kidney tissue. Can also be genetically determined or caused by other metabolic disorders.

Polyuria
Abnormally increased urine output of more than 3 liters per day. Also occurs in other conditions such as diabetes.

2. 2. 3. Monitoring of Vitamin D Levels

egular monitoring of vitamin D levels is crucial for the safety and success of therapy during high-dose supplementation. Systematic monitoring allows for optimal dose adjustment and minimizes potential risks. After initiating a high-dose therapy or after any dose adjustment, the first follow-up appointment should occur after three months [s122]. This provides the body with sufficient time to reach a new equilibrium. A practical example: If a patient begins high-dose vitamin D3 therapy in January, the first check should take place in April. In addition to the vitamin D level (25-OHD), other important laboratory parameters must be monitored. These include calcium, phosphorus, and albumin levels [s122]. These values provide important insights into possible side effects or metabolic changes. A documentation sheet that records all measurements chronologically helps to identify trends early. For long-term monitoring, a seasonal check-up schedule has proven effective: A measurement in spring shows the lower values after winter, while an autumn measurement reflects the higher values after summer [s123]. The supplementation dose can then be adjusted accordingly. For example, the dose could be increased in winter and reduced in summer.

For patients with chronic kidney disease (CKD), specific monitoring intervals apply [s124]:
- CKD Stage G3a-G3b: Calcium and phosphate every 6-12 months
- CKD Stage G4: Calcium and phosphate every 3-6 months, <u>PTH</u> every 6-12 months
- CKD Stage G5: Calcium and phosphate every 1-3 months, PTH every 3-6 months

Particularly close monitoring is required for high-risk patients, such as those with <u>malabsorption syndromes</u> or kidney failure [s125]. In these cases, monitoring should be conducted by a specialist. A monitoring calendar that includes all upcoming appointments can help patients avoid missing important tests.

After a <u>bolus therapy</u> with very high doses of vitamin D, a specific monitoring protocol must be followed [s126]:
- Serum calcium check after 1-2 weeks
- Vitamin D measurement after 1 month
- Comprehensive check after 3 months

Therapeutic decisions should never be based solely on individual laboratory values but should always consider trends and all available parameters [s124]. For example, if the vitamin D level is within the target range but serum calcium is continuously rising, a dose reduction may be necessary.

Practical recommendations for patients:
- Keep a "Vitamin D diary" with all intakes and measurements
- Use reminder functions on your smartphone for follow-up appointments
- Educate yourself about typical symptoms of overdose
- Bring a current overview of your measurements to each doctor's appointment

If the 25-OHD level remains below 30 ng/mL despite two bolus therapies, an <u>endocrinological</u> evaluation is indicated [s122]. This could indicate underlying metabolic disorders or absorption issues.

Glossary

Bolus Therapy
A short-term treatment with very high doses of a medication to quickly achieve a therapeutic effect.

Endocrinological
Refers to the medical specialty that deals with hormones and hormone-producing organs.

Malabsorption Syndrome
A group of disorders where nutrient absorption in the intestine is impaired, potentially leading to deficiencies.

PTH
Parathyroid hormone - a hormone from the parathyroid glands that regulates calcium and phosphate balance.

2. 2. 4. Possible Interactions with Medications

n the case of high-dose vitamin D3 supplementation, various drug interactions must be considered, as these can affect the efficacy of the therapy or lead to undesirable side effects. A careful coordination between the treating physician and the patient is therefore essential. Particularly relevant are interactions with enzyme inducers, which can influence vitamin D metabolism [s127]. This includes antiepileptic drugs such as carbamazepine, phenytoin, and oxcarbazepine. A patient taking these medications may require a higher vitamin D3 dose to achieve therapeutic levels. Treating physicians should closely monitor vitamin D levels in such cases. Significant changes in plasma levels can also occur with the simultaneous intake of HIV medications, especially protease inhibitors and non-nucleoside reverse transcriptase inhibitors [s127]. A practical example: An HIV patient undergoing antiretroviral therapy should closely coordinate their vitamin D3 supplementation with their treating physician and undergo regular level checks. Particular caution is warranted when taking herbal preparations. For instance, St. John's Wort can act as an enzyme inducer, accelerating the metabolism of vitamin D3 [s127]. Patients should therefore discuss all supplements and herbal preparations with their doctor. The interactions between vitamin D3 and cholesterol-lowering medications deserve special attention. High doses of vitamin D3 can reduce the effectiveness of certain statins [s128]. A practical tip: Take vitamin D3 and cholesterol-lowering medications at different times of the day to minimize potential interactions. For patients taking anticoagulants, attention to vitamin K levels is important. Although vitamin D3 itself does not directly interact with anticoagulants, altered vitamin K intake can influence the effect of blood thinners [s128].

Practical recommendations for patients undergoing high-dose vitamin D3 therapy:
- Maintain a complete list of all medications taken, including herbal preparations
- Inform all treating physicians about the high-dose vitamin D3 therapy
- Adhere to established dosing times, especially in known interactions
- Document unusual symptoms or side effects
- Avoid self-adjusting doses

The labeling of high-dose vitamin D3 preparations contains important warnings about possible interactions [s129]. This information should be read and considered carefully. A structured medication plan that accounts for all dosing times and potential interactions can help enhance therapy safety. In complex medication regimens, especially in older patients or those with multiple underlying conditions, pharmaceutical consultation is recommended. The pharmacist can identify potential interactions and provide practical recommendations for the timing of doses. Regular review of the medication by the treating physician is essential, as interactions often only manifest during the course of therapy. Over-the-counter medications and supplements should also be considered, as these can influence vitamin D metabolism.

Glossary

Anticoagulant
Medications that inhibit blood clotting and are used to prevent thrombosis.

Enzyme Inducer
A substance that increases the formation of certain enzymes in the liver, thereby accelerating the breakdown of medications.

Protease Inhibitor
Medications that block certain enzymes (proteases) and are primarily used in HIV therapy.

Statin
Medications used to lower cholesterol levels by inhibiting a specific enzyme in the liver.

Summary - 2. 2. High-dose Vitamin D3 Supplementation

- 50% of US children aged 1-5 years and 70% of those aged 6-11 years exhibit a vitamin D deficiency.
- Patients with Crohn's disease often require three to four times the usual supplementation dose.
- After bariatric procedures, a minimum of 3000 IU daily is recommended to achieve a target level of 28 ng/mL.
- In cases of hypercalcemia due to overdose, the risk is 4 cases per 1000 individuals at 3200-4000 IU daily.
- The safe upper intake limit for children aged 1-10 years is 50 micrograms daily.
- A 25-hydroxyvitamin D level above 125 nmol/L is considered too high.
- After the initiation of therapy or dose adjustment, the first follow-up should occur after three months.
- In chronic kidney disease stage G5, calcium and phosphate levels should be monitored every 1-3 months.
- After a loading therapy, serum calcium must be checked after 1-2 weeks.
- Antiepileptics such as carbamazepine can influence vitamin D metabolism through enzyme induction.
- HIV medications, especially protease inhibitors, can significantly alter plasma vitamin D levels.
- St. John's Wort accelerates the metabolism of vitamin D3 as an enzyme inducer.

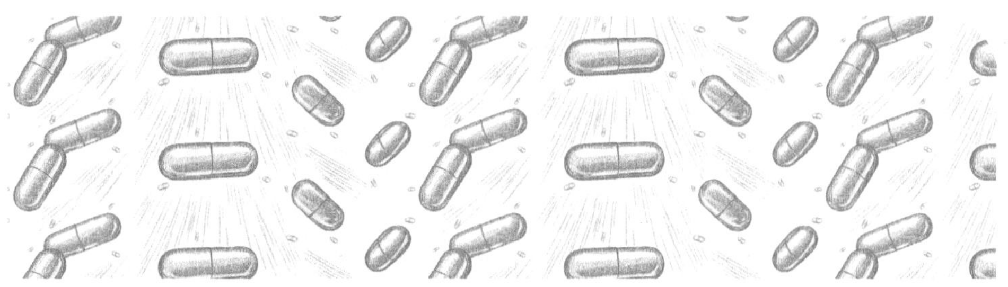

2. 3. Forms of Intake and Timing

he correct intake of Vitamin D3 raises fundamental questions for many people: Which form of administration is best suited? When is the optimal time for intake? Should the supplement be taken with or without a meal? And what role does the combination with other nutrients, such as Vitamin K2, play? The choice of the appropriate form of intake and the right timing can significantly influence the effectiveness of Vitamin D3 supplementation. Not only personal preferences matter, but also scientific findings regarding the bioavailability of different forms of administration and optimal absorption in the body. The following sections provide evidence-based answers to these important questions and outline practical ways to optimize your Vitamin D3 supplementation.

„Vitamin D3 can still have positive effects on the body's levels two years after ingestion."

2. 3. 1. Tablets, Capsules, and Drops

itamin D3 is available in various forms, each offering specific advantages and disadvantages [s130]. The most commonly used forms are tablets, capsules, and drops, with the D3 form (cholecalciferol) being preferred due to its more efficient absorption in the small intestine [s131]. Oily drop solutions exhibit particularly high bioverfuegbarkeit compared to solid forms [s131]. This makes them especially interesting for individuals with absorption disorders or digestive issues. A practical tip for taking vitamin D3 drops: place them directly on a spoon and preferably take them with a fatty meal, as this further enhances absorption. Soft capsules represent another popular option, as they already contain vitamin D3 in an oily solution. They are particularly convenient for on-the-go use and allow for precise dosing. For individuals with swallowing difficulties, the capsules can also be carefully punctured, and the contents expressed. An innovative development is orodispersible films (ODFs), which dissolve quickly in the mouth and do not require water for ingestion [s131]. This form is especially suitable for children and the elderly, as it is easy to take and has high acceptance. The rapid dissolution in the mouth also leads to quicker release of the active ingredient. Dosage varies depending on age group and individual needs. While a daily dose of 600 IU is sufficient for most healthy adults, individuals over 70 years require about 800 IU daily [s132]. Infants should receive between 200 and 400 IU in their first year of life [s132]. A practical aspect of vitamin D3 supplementation is the possibility of weekly or monthly intake, as the active ingredient accumulates in fat tissue and is released as needed [s131]. For individuals with fat absorption issues, lactose intolerance, or milk allergies, supplementation is particularly important [s132]. In these cases, the use of drops or special soft capsules that ensure optimal absorption is recommended. When selecting the appropriate form of administration, individual factors such as swallowing ability, preferences, and any accompanying health conditions should be considered. A practical tip is to integrate the intake into the daily routine, for example, at breakfast or dinner, to avoid forgetting regular consumption. The storage of the preparations should be cool, dry, and protected from light. Especially with drops, attention should be paid to the limited shelf life after opening. A practical note: mark the opening date on the bottle to keep track of its shelf life. Vitamin D3 is initially stored in fat cells after ingestion and remains inactive there until the body needs it [s132]. Activation occurs through hydroxylation in the liver and kidneys [s132], ensuring a continuous supply even if intake does not occur daily.

Glossary

Absorption Disorder
Impairment of nutrient absorption in the digestive tract, often caused by intestinal diseases

Hydroxylation
Chemical process in which a hydroxyl group (OH) is attached to a molecule, important for the activation of vitamins

Orodispersible
A form of medication that dissolves in the mouth without the addition of water and can be absorbed through the oral mucosa

2. 3. 2. Optimal Timing of Intake

The choice of the optimal timing for Vitamin D3 intake is influenced by both seasonal and daily factors. Particularly during the autumn and winter months, regular supplementation is recommended, as the body's own Vitamin D production through sunlight is significantly reduced during this time [s133]. For most individuals, year-round supplementation is sensible, especially if they spend little time outdoors. The recommendation is a daily dose of 10 micrograms (400 IU) for adults and children over 4 years [s133]. A practical approach is to integrate the intake into the morning routine, as this supports the natural biorhythm. For instance, set an alarm on your smartphone to remind you to take it at the same time each day. Special attention should be given to the seasonal adjustment of supplementation. While from the end of March to the end of September, most people can meet their Vitamin D needs through sunlight and diet, consistent supplementation is important during the darker months [s133]. For athletes and individuals living at higher latitudes, the winter period is particularly critical. They should be especially diligent with their supplementation during this time [s134]. A practical tip for dose adjustment: Keep a simple "sun diary" in which you document your daily sunlight exposure. This helps you better assess the necessity of supplementation. Individuals who work shifts or predominantly indoors should also supplement during the summer. Specific recommendations apply to certain population groups. Pregnant and breastfeeding women should pay particular attention to adequate supply, especially during the winter months [s133]. Children aged 1 to 4 years require a daily intake of 10 micrograms of Vitamin D year-round [s133]. It is advisable to associate the Vitamin D intake with a regular meal, such as breakfast. In therapeutic applications, such as supporting recovery, higher dosages like 5000 IU daily over a defined period of about two weeks may be sensible [s135]. However, such higher dosages should only be taken after consulting with medical professionals. Another practical aspect is coordinating Vitamin D intake with other supplements or medications. Create a clear intake schedule if you are taking multiple preparations. For example, Vitamin D3 can be well taken at breakfast, ideally along with a fatty meal. For individuals with irregular daily routines, it may be helpful to associate Vitamin D intake with another daily habit, such as brushing teeth or having morning coffee. Set realistic times for intake and remain flexible – it is more important to take the supplement regularly than to adhere to an exact timing. Also, consider the importance of long-term planning: At the beginning of the autumn/winter season, ensure you have an adequate supply of Vitamin D3. This helps avoid supply gaps due to forgotten repurchases. A practical tip is to set a reminder in your calendar when your supply is running low.

2. 3. 3. Intake with or without meals

he intake of Vitamin D3 in conjunction with meals plays an important role in optimal absorption in the body. Interestingly, recent studies show that a low-fat meal promotes the absorption of Vitamin D3 more effectively than a high-fat meal or intake without food [s136]. This contradicts the long-held assumption that a high-fat meal is the best option. Specifically, research has found that Vitamin D3 levels rose significantly higher within 12 hours after intake with a low-fat meal compared to other forms of intake [s136]. A practical example of a suitable low-fat meal would be a light breakfast with whole grain bread, lean cold cuts, and some vegetables. Avoid very fatty components such as butter, cheese, or high-fat sausages. The intake recommendations may vary depending on the preparation. While some forms, such as calcium citrate, can be taken flexibly with or without meals, other preparations, such as calcium carbonate, should preferably be taken during a meal [s137]. This underscores the importance of carefully reading the package insert or consulting a doctor or pharmacist. To monitor the effectiveness of supplementation, it is advisable to have the Vitamin D level determined before starting intake and to conduct a follow-up measurement after about three months [s138]. This allows for individual adjustment of dosage and intake schedule. A practical tip: Keep a calendar where you document both regular intake and the dates for blood tests. For practical implementation in daily life, it is advisable to associate Vitamin D3 intake with a regular meal. For example, choose breakfast or lunch as a fixed intake time. Prepare your portion for the upcoming week in a pill organizer and place it visibly next to your eating area. When taking multiple supplements or medications, potential interactions should be considered. Create a clear intake plan that takes into account the optimal intervals between different preparations. A reminder function on your smartphone can also be helpful, alerting you to take your supplements at the right time. For people with irregular meal times, such as shift workers, it is particularly important to develop a practical routine. One option would be to take the Vitamin D3 preparation always with the first larger meal of the day, regardless of the time. It is important that the meal is not too high in fat to ensure optimal absorption. The regularity of intake is more important than the exact timing. Therefore, develop a routine that fits your personal daily schedule. If, for example, you often skip breakfast, lunch might be the better time for intake.

The main thing is that you take the preparation regularly and in conjunction with an appropriate meal.

2. 3. 4. Combination with Vitamin K2

he combination of Vitamin D3 with Vitamin K2 is gaining increasing importance in modern supplementation. Scientific studies demonstrate that these two vitamins work synergistically and support each other in their functionality [s139]. Particularly important is the role of Vitamin K2, which is considered a crucial factor in directing calcium specifically into the bones while simultaneously preventing unwanted deposits in the arteries [s140]. Taking high-dose Vitamin D3 without sufficient K2 supply can even pose health risks [s140]. A practical approach is therefore the use of combination preparations that contain both vitamins in a balanced ratio. These are available in both tablet and liquid form [s141]. For optimal effectiveness, a daily dose of at least 90 micrograms of Vitamin K2 has proven effective, especially in postmenopausal women for reducing bone loss [s142]. A practical tip for everyday life: When purchasing Vitamin D3 preparations, ensure that they are already enriched with K2, or supplement your intake accordingly. Particularly interesting are the research findings in diabetes patients. The combined intake of both vitamins led to a significant improvement in blood sugar levels and insulin sensitivity [s143]. Therefore, it is advisable for diabetics to discuss supplementation with their treating physician and, if necessary, monitor blood sugar levels more closely. The combination of Vitamin K2 with calcium and Vitamin D3 shows particularly positive effects on the bone density of the lumbar spine [s144]. A practical approach here would be to combine supplementation with a calcium-rich breakfast in the morning. For example, one could take the vitamins with a muesli containing almonds and calcium-fortified plant milk. For the long-term health of bones and the cardiovascular system, the balanced combination of both vitamins is of great importance [s140]. There are no known risks associated with simultaneous intake—in fact, the combination is considered safer than the sole intake of Vitamin D3 [s141]. A practical tip for implementation: Create a supplementation plan that considers both vitamins. For instance, use a weekly pill organizer and combine intake with a regular meal. Additionally, document your intake and any changes in a health diary. For individuals at increased risk for osteoporosis or cardiovascular diseases, combined supplementation is particularly relevant [s140]. A practical approach would be to have regular bone density measurements conducted and adjust supplementation accordingly. The choice of the right K2 form is also significant, as different forms have varying half-lives in the body [s140]. It is advisable to consult a nutrition expert or physician who can consider your individual situation. For optimal absorption of both vitamins, it is recommended to take them together with a light, not overly fatty meal. A practical example would be a light breakfast with whole grain bread and lean protein, complemented by vitamin K2-rich foods such as fermented products.

synergistic
Describes the interaction of various factors, where the overall effect is greater than the sum of the individual effects - like two musicians who sound better together than alone.

2. 3. 5. Storage and Shelf Life of Supplements

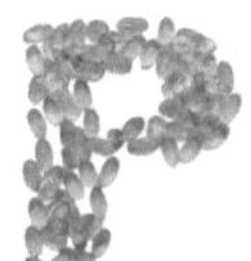

roper storage of Vitamin D3 supplements is crucial for their effectiveness and shelf life. Scientific studies show that the stability of the vitamin is influenced by various environmental factors [s145]. Protection from direct sunlight, heat, and moisture is particularly important. Liquid Vitamin D3 supplements require special attention when stored. In aqueous solutions, Vitamin D3 is very unstable—its concentration in distilled water drops to below 10% of the original content after just one day at room temperature [s145]. A practical tip: Store drop formulations in the refrigerator after opening and note the opening date on the bottle. The chemical stability of Vitamin D3 is significantly affected by the pH value. The vitamin is most stable at a pH above 5, while it rapidly degrades under acidic conditions (pH 1-4) [s145]. In practice, this means: Avoid taking Vitamin D3 supplements together with acidic beverages like fruit juices. For prescription liquid formulations, manufacturers ensure that the active ingredient content remains above 90% of the declared value for at least one year at 25°C and four months at 40°C through overdosing [s146]. Therefore, a cool place with a constant temperature, such as a medicine cabinet in the bedroom, is recommended for home storage. Exposure to oxygen significantly reduces the stability of Vitamin D3 [s145]. A practical piece of advice: Close the supplements carefully immediately after each use and avoid frequently opening the packaging. For drop bottles, it is advisable to store them upside down so that the dropper remains moistened and does not dry out. Interestingly, Vitamin D3 can still have positive effects on the body's levels even two years after ingestion [s147]. This underscores the importance of proper storage to ensure this long-term effect. For household organization, it is advisable to follow a "First-in-First-out" approach: Place new packages at the back and older ones at the front. The presence of certain metal ions such as iron(II), copper(I), and copper(II) accelerates the degradation of Vitamin D3, with iron(II) having the strongest negative effect [s145]. Practical consequence: Do not store Vitamin D3 supplements together with iron-containing supplements and avoid metallic storage containers. For measuring the Vitamin D status in the body, it is reassuring to know that 25(OH)D is very stable under common laboratory conditions: 4 hours at room temperature, 24 hours at 2-8°C, 7 days at -20°C, and even 3 months at -80°C [s148]. For patients, this means that blood samples can provide reliable results even after longer transport times. A practical system for monitoring shelf life: Create a simple table with all Vitamin D3 supplements in the household, noting the purchase date, opening date, and expiration date. Check the entries monthly and dispose of expired supplements properly.

Glossary

pH value

A measure of the concentration of hydrogen ions in a solution, indicated on a scale from 0 (very acidic) to 14 (very basic), with 7 being neutral.

Summary - 2. 3. Forms of Intake and Timing

- Oily drop solutions show the highest bioavailability for Vitamin D3. Orodispersible films dissolve quickly in the mouth and allow for rapid release of the active ingredient. The activation of Vitamin D3 occurs through hydroxylation in the liver and kidneys. Contrary to previous assumptions, a low-fat meal promotes absorption more than a high-fat meal. Vitamin D3 levels significantly increase within 12 hours after ingestion with a low-fat meal. The combination of D3 with K2 prevents unwanted calcium deposits in the arteries. 90 micrograms of Vitamin K2 daily demonstrably reduce bone loss in postmenopausal women. The D3/K2 combination improves blood sugar levels and insulin sensitivity in diabetics. In aqueous solutions, the D3 concentration falls below 10% after one day at room temperature. Vitamin D3 is most stable at pH values above 5. Iron(II) ions accelerate the degradation of Vitamin D3 the most. 25(OH)D remains stable for 7 days at -20°C and for 3 months at -80°C.

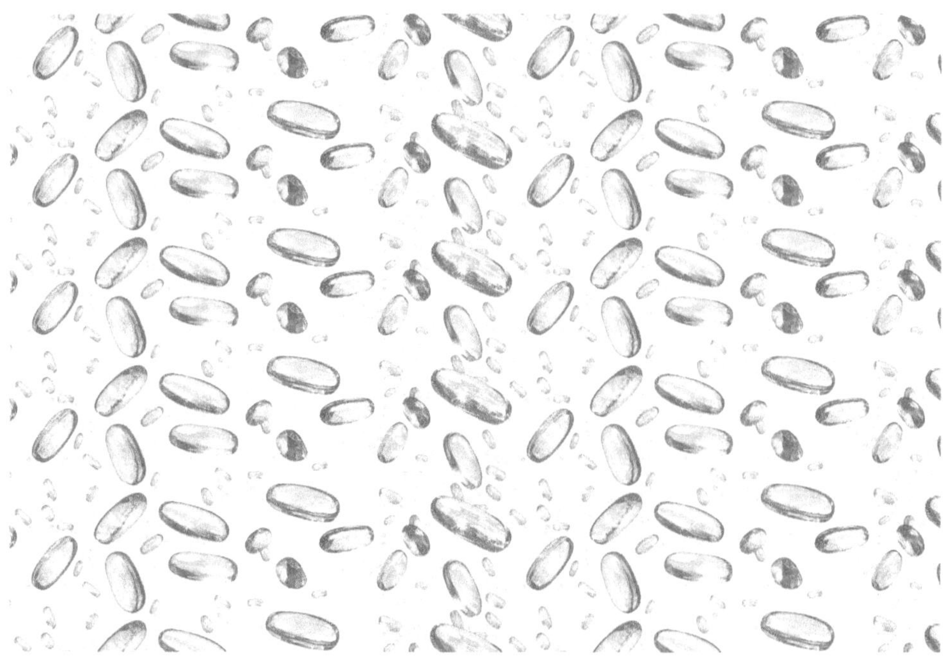

Review - 2. Dosage and Application of Vitamin D3

- The recommended daily dose for adults aged 19-70 years is 600 IU, which increases to 800 IU from the age of 71.
- Recent research suggests higher doses of 1500-2000 IU for an optimal 25-hydroxyvitamin D level of at least 30 ng/mL.
- The safe upper intake limit is 4000 IU per day, with studies indicating that even 5000 IU does not cause serious side effects.
- In cases of malabsorption syndromes and after bariatric procedures, a minimum of 3000 IU daily is recommended.
- High-dose vitamin D3 supplementation without adequate K2 intake may pose health risks.
- The combination with vitamin K2 (at least 90 micrograms daily) is particularly effective in reducing bone loss in postmenopausal women.
- In aqueous solutions, vitamin D3 is very unstable—the concentration drops to below 10% after just one day at room temperature.
- Chemical stability is significantly influenced by pH, with vitamin D3 being most stable at a pH above 5.
- Vitamin D3 can still have positive effects on body levels even two years after ingestion.
- The presence of metal ions such as iron(II), copper(I), and copper(II) accelerates the degradation of vitamin D3.
- While these facts are essential for correct dosing and application, they raise the intriguing question of what specific health benefits optimal vitamin D3 supply actually offers.

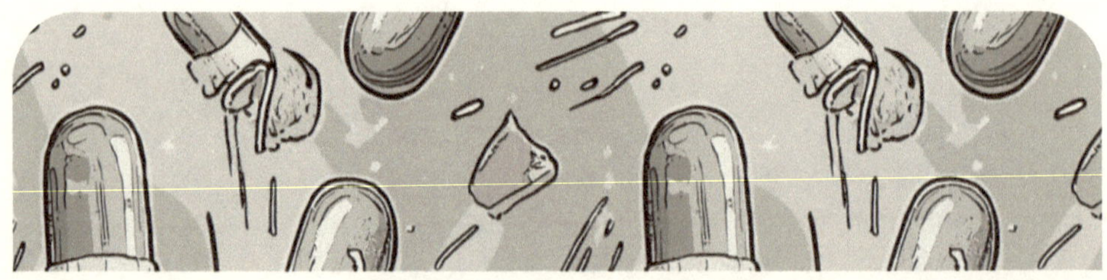

3. Effects and Benefits of Vitamin D3 Supplementation

he effects and benefits of optimal vitamin D3 supply extend far beyond the classical bone metabolism. While its fundamental importance for healthy bones has long been known, current research increasingly demonstrates how profoundly this vitamin influences our health. But what mechanisms underlie its diverse effects? How exactly does vitamin D3 support our immune system in defending against pathogens? In recent years, science has uncovered surprising connections between vitamin D3 levels and the function of various organ systems. From the modulation of immune responses to the regulation of inflammatory processes, these findings raise new questions: What role does vitamin D3 play in the prevention of autoimmune diseases? How can its immunomodulatory effects be therapeutically utilized? The following sections illuminate the scientific foundations and practical aspects of vitamin D3 supplementation. They reveal how this fascinating vitamin affects our health at the molecular level and what concrete benefits optimal supply offers.

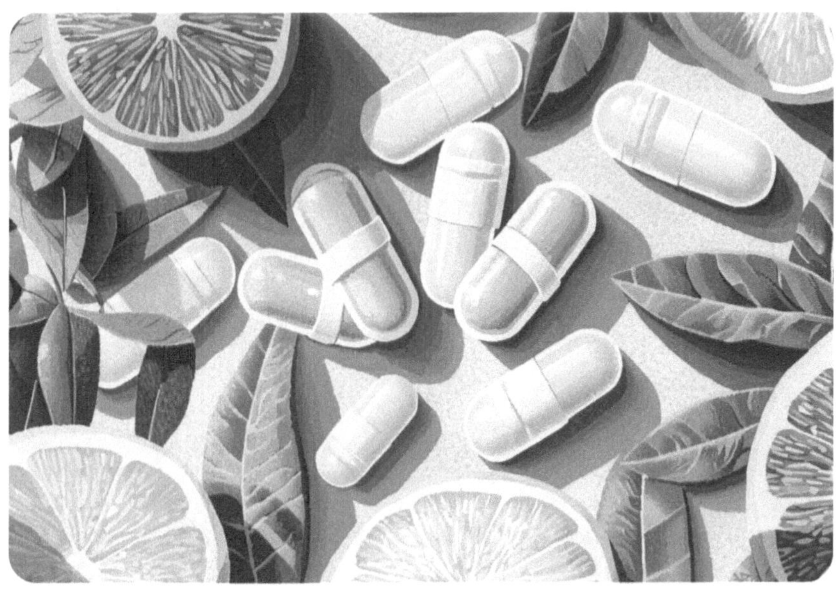

3. 1. Bone Health and Osteoporosis Prevention

he importance of healthy bones for our quality of life often becomes apparent only when problems arise. But how does bone strength actually develop over the course of our lives? What role does Vitamin D3 play in maintaining bone health, and why is adequate supply particularly important during childhood? Research over the past decades has shown that bone health depends on a complex interplay of various factors. This raises the question of how we can keep our bones healthy into old age through targeted measures. Which preventive strategies are scientifically proven, and how can they be integrated into daily life? The following sections illuminate the fascinating mechanisms of bone strengthening and demonstrate how Vitamin D3, along with other nutrients, sustainably supports our bone health.

„The highest bone density is reached by humans between the ages of 25 and 35.“

3. 1. 1. Mechanism of Bone Strengthening

uman bone is an astonishingly dynamic tissue that undergoes a continuous process of renewal [s149]. This complex mechanism of bone strengthening is based on the balanced interplay of various cell types and metabolic processes that interlock like a precise clockwork. At the center of this process are two main players: the bone-forming osteoblasts and the bone-resorbing osteoclasts [s150]. Imagine these cells as a team of construction workers—while osteoblasts build new bone material, osteoclasts remove old or damaged tissue. This balance is crucial for the health of our bones. Humans achieve peak bone density between the ages of 25 and 35 [s151]. This underscores the importance of investing in bone health at a young age. A practical tip: those who engage in regular exercise and maintain a balanced diet during this life stage essentially establish a "bone account" for later years.

Calcium plays a key role as a building block for healthy bones [s152]. Interestingly, our body only absorbs 15-20% of the calcium ingested [s151]. To optimize this absorption, vitamin D3 is essential. It acts like a key that opens the door to improved calcium uptake. A practical everyday tip: combine calcium-rich foods with a short walk in the sun, as our body can produce vitamin D3 through sunlight [s153]. Vitamin K complements this interplay perfectly by increasing bone density and reducing fracture risk [s154]. It activates specific proteins such as osteocalcin, which are indispensable for

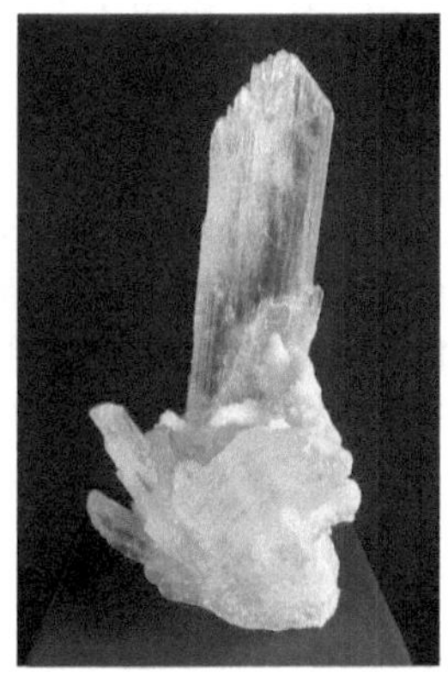

Calcium [i10]

bone mineralization. In practice, this means that a diet rich in green leafy vegetables, which contain plenty of vitamin K, actively supports your bone health.

The vitamin D receptor (VDR) plays a central role in gene regulation for calcium and phosphate metabolism [s155]. It acts like a conductor coordinating the orchestra of bone cells. In doing so, it activates the production of <u>osteoprotegerin</u> (OPG) and inhibits <u>RANKL</u>, which slows down bone resorption. As we age, this delicate mechanism changes. Kidney function declines, which impairs vitamin D activation [s156]. At the same time, calcium absorption in the intestine decreases. A

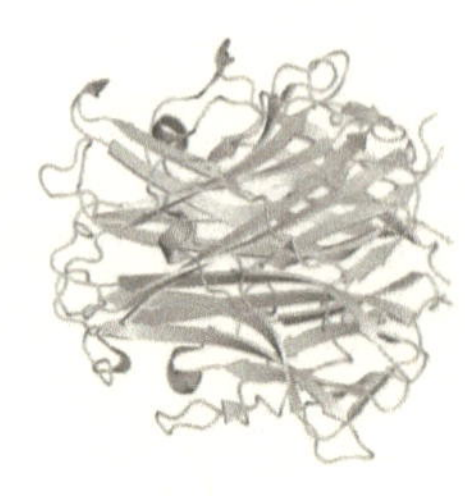

RANKL [i11]

practical piece of advice for older individuals: regularly check your vitamin D levels and discuss potential supplementation with your doctor. Estrogen plays a particularly important role in bone health for women [s157]. After menopause, when estrogen levels drop, the risk of osteoporosis increases. An active lifestyle with regular exercise can counteract this. Practical exercises such as climbing stairs or moderate strength training are effective measures for strengthening bones. Inflammatory processes can accelerate bone resorption [s157]. Therefore, it is important to avoid inflammatory factors such as smoking [s151]. A balanced lifestyle with adequate sleep and stress management further supports bone health. For optimal vitamin D supply, experts recommend sensible sun exposure of 5-10 minutes for arms and legs or face, 2-3 times a week [s153]. This should be combined with a balanced diet rich in calcium, vitamin D, and protein [s151].

Osteoblast

Specialized bone cells that arise from stem cells and form new bone substance through the production of collagen and other proteins.

Osteocalcin

A protein produced by osteoblasts that binds calcium and is important for the formation of hydroxyapatite crystals in bone.

Osteoclast

Multinucleated giant cells that can dissolve old bone tissue through the secretion of acids and enzymes.

Osteoprotegerin

A protein that acts as a natural protective mechanism against excessive bone resorption by blocking the RANKL signaling pathway.

RANKL

A signaling molecule that regulates the development and activation of bone-resorbing cells and can lead to bone loss when activity is increased.

3. 1. 2. Reduction of Fracture Risk

The reduction of fracture risk requires a holistic approach that combines various preventive measures. Scientific studies impressively demonstrate that the combined supplementation of calcium and vitamin D can reduce the overall fracture risk by 15% and the specific risk of hip fractures by as much as 30% [s158]. This finding is particularly relevant for older adults, as approximately one-third of individuals over 65 fall at least once a year, with 5-6% of these falls resulting in fractures [s159]. A crucial component of fracture prevention is the regular assessment of vitamin D status through the measurement of the plasma 25(OH)D level [s160]. This is especially important for individuals with an increased fracture risk or existing bone diseases. As a guideline, values below 25 nmol/L indicate a deficiency, while values between 25-50 nmol/L are often considered insufficient [s160]. A practical tip for daily life: Have your vitamin D levels regularly checked by your general practitioner, especially during the sun-poor winter months. The optimal dosage of vitamin D plays a decisive role. Studies show that a daily intake of 800-1000 ie of vitamin D can reduce the risk of falls by a remarkable 22% [s159]. Interestingly, regular daily intake is more effective than sporadic high-dose therapy. It is important to note that very high doses of vitamin D can paradoxically increase the risk of falls and fractures in the first months after intake [s160]. For postmenopausal women and men over 50 who exhibit an increased risk of osteoporosis or fractures, a balanced, nutrient-rich diet is of particular importance [s161]. A practical dietary plan could include daily components such as low-fat dairy products, leafy green vegetables, fatty fish, and whole grains. A key aspect of fracture prevention is systematic fall assessment [s161]. This should be conducted for all patients with osteoporosis or previous fractures. Various risk factors such as vision, medication, home environment, and mobility are evaluated. A practical tip: Remove tripping hazards in your home, such as loose rugs or cables, and ensure adequate lighting. The guidelines for osteoporosis prevention recommend a comprehensive risk assessment for individuals with clinical risk factors for fragilitaetsfrakturen [s162]. This includes measuring bone density and, if necessary, further examinations. An important practical note: Create a list of your personal risk factors with your doctor, such as family history, medication use, or previous fractures [s163]. Fracture prevention requires an integrated care approach [s162]. This includes not only pharmacological therapy but also targeted exercise programs to improve strength and balance. An effective exercise program could consist of a combination of Tai Chi for balance, light strength training for muscles, and regular walking. A large meta-analysis involving over 30,970 participants confirms the effectiveness of combined supplementation of minerals and vitamins for fracture prevention [s164]. This scientific evidence underscores the importance of a holistic prevention strategy that encompasses nutrition, exercise, and, if necessary, supplementation.

3. 1. 3. Interaction with Calcium

he complex interplay between calcium and other nutrients in the body resembles a finely tuned orchestra. Calcium, as the most abundant mineral in the human body, is stored 99% in our bones and teeth [s165]. However, the optimal utilization of this essential mineral depends on various factors. Calcium metabolism does not function in isolation; rather, it is the result of a sophisticated collaboration between calcium, phosphorus, vitamin D, and proteins [s165]. For instance, if vitamin D is lacking, the body responds with an increased production of parathormon (PTH), which in turn accelerates bone resorption and increases the risk of osteoporosis [s166]. A practical tip for daily life: When taking calcium supplements, always ensure adequate vitamin D intake to guarantee optimal absorption and utilization. Interestingly, microorganisms in our gut also play a significant role in calcium absorption [s167]. The gut microbiota influences, through various mechanisms, how well minerals from food can be absorbed. A crucial factor in this process is the reduction of pH levels in the gut [s167]. To support these natural processes, regular consumption of fermented dairy products is recommended. These not only contain calcium but also beneficial probiotics, which have been shown to reduce age-related bone loss [s168]. Solely taking calcium supplements is often insufficient for osteoporosis prevention and can, in some cases, even be counterproductive [s169]. New research shows promising results for the combination of calcium with chondroitin sulfate. This combination can increase bone density and improve calcium concentration specifically in the femur [s169]. A practical approach would be to ensure calcium intake from various sources: for example, a natural yogurt with berries in the morning, a portion of leafy greens at lunch, and a glass of fermented buttermilk in the evening.

The interactions between gut bacteria and minerals can also influence the production of hormones that regulate calcium metabolism [s167]. A healthy gut microbiome thus indirectly contributes to bone health. Practical measures to promote a healthy gut flora include:
- Regular consumption of fermented foods such as kefir, yogurt, or sauerkraut
- A fiber-rich diet with plenty of vegetables and whole grains
- Avoiding excessive sugar and alcohol consumption

Probiotics can help improve mineral balance and prevent disturbances in parathyroid hormone levels [s168]. A balanced ratio of gut bacteria not only supports calcium absorption but can also mitigate age-related increases in <u>bone resorption</u> [s168]. A practical tip: Combine calcium-rich foods with probiotic products, for example, in the form of a muesli with yogurt and calcium-rich nuts. Optimal calcium supply is thus a complex interplay of various factors, where, in addition to pure calcium intake, gut health, vitamin D supply, and other nutrients play a crucial role. A holistic approach to bone health should consider all these aspects.

Glossary

Bone Resorption

The natural breakdown of bone tissue by specialized cells (osteoclasts). This process is part of normal bone remodeling but can become excessive in cases of disturbance.

Chondroitin Sulfate

A natural component of cartilage tissue used as a dietary supplement. It supports the formation and maintenance of cartilage substance.

Microbiota

The totality of all microorganisms that inhabit the human gut. It consists of over 100 trillion bacteria and more than 1000 different species.

Probiotics

Live microorganisms that have positive health effects when consumed in adequate amounts. They can colonize the gut and support the natural balance of gut flora.

3. 1. 4. Prevention of Rickets in Children

The prevention of <u>rickets</u> in children is an important health issue that can be completely avoided through targeted measures [s170]. This condition, which impairs bone development in children, can be effectively prevented by ensuring adequate vitamin D supply. Particularly important is prevention during pregnancy. Expectant mothers should take 600-1000 IU of vitamin D daily [s170] [s171]. This is comparable to a 20-30 minute walk on a sunny day, with the face and arms exposed to the sun. A practical tip for pregnant women: Incorporate a "vitamin D walk" into your daily routine, preferably in the morning or early afternoon. Special recommendations apply to newborns and infants. Breastfed infants should receive 400-800 IU of vitamin D daily during the first year of life [s170] [s171]. This is especially important as breast milk alone does not provide sufficient vitamin D [s172]. A practical piece of advice for breastfeeding mothers: Place the vitamin D drops for the baby next to the breastfeeding supplies to avoid forgetting the daily dose. For infants fed with formula, an additional supplementation of 400 IU of vitamin D per day is recommended [s171]. This is in addition to the vitamin D already present in the infant formula. Parents should ideally associate the vitamin D administration with a fixed daily routine, such as with the morning bottle. Special recommendations apply to premature infants: They require 400 IU of vitamin D and 150-220 mg/kg of calcium daily [s173]. This increased intake is important as premature infants are particularly susceptible to vitamin D deficiency. A practical tip for parents of premature infants: Keep a nutrition diary to monitor daily vitamin and mineral intake. As children grow older, the recommendations change. Children aged 1 to 18 years should consume 600 IU of vitamin D and 600-800 mg of calcium daily [s173]. This can be supported by a balanced diet and regular outdoor activity. A concrete suggestion: Establish "outdoor playtimes," ideally between 10 AM and 3 PM, when UV radiation is optimal for the body's vitamin D production. In at-risk groups, such as children with limited sun exposure or <u>malabsorption disorders</u>, higher doses of 400-1000 IU of vitamin D daily may be necessary [s173]. In such cases, regular monitoring of vitamin D levels by the pediatrician is particularly important. In cases of existing vitamin D deficiency, intensified therapy is necessary. Affected children then require 2000 IU daily or 50,000 IU weekly over a period of 6 weeks [s174]. Subsequently, a maintenance therapy of 1000 IU daily is implemented. The prevention of rickets requires a holistic approach that considers nutrition, supplementation, and lifestyle [s170]. Parents should work closely with their pediatrician and attend regular check-ups. A practical tip: Create a "prevention calendar" that includes appointments for check-ups, vitamin D supplementation, and regular outdoor activities.

Glossary

Malabsorption

A disorder of nutrient absorption in the intestine, which can have various causes, such as celiac disease or chronic inflammatory bowel diseases.

Rickets

A condition characterized by insufficient mineralization of the bone, which can lead to skeletal deformities. Typical signs include bow legs, knock knees, and delayed development of the fontanelle.

Summary - 3. 1. Bone Health and Osteoporosis Prevention

- The highest bone density is reached between the ages of 25 and 35.
- The body absorbs only 15-20% of the calcium ingested.
- The vitamin D receptor (VDR) regulates calcium and phosphate metabolism through gene regulation.
- Osteoprotegerin (OPG) and RANKL are key factors in controlling bone resorption.
- Combined supplementation of calcium and vitamin D reduces the overall fracture risk by 15% and the hip fracture risk by 30%.
- About one-third of individuals over 65 fall at least once a year, with 5-6% of these falls resulting in fractures.
- A daily intake of 800-1000 IU of vitamin D reduces the fall risk by 22%.
- The gut microbiota influences mineral absorption by lowering the pH in the intestine.
- Chondroitin sulfate combined with calcium specifically improves bone density in the femur.
- Probiotics can mitigate age-related increases in bone resorption.
- Premature infants require 400 IU of vitamin D and 150-220 mg/kg of calcium daily.
- In cases of vitamin D deficiency, an intensive therapy of 2000 IU daily or 50,000 IU weekly for 6 weeks is necessary.

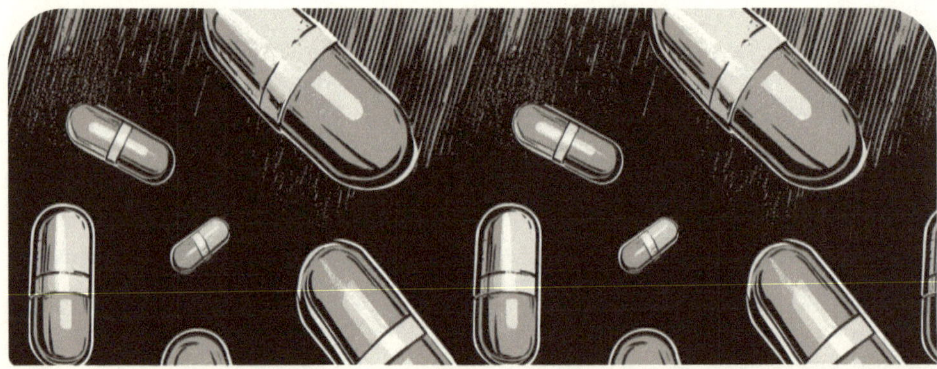

3. 2. Immune System and Infection Defense

he role of the immune system in defending against pathogens is fundamentally important for our health. But how exactly does Vitamin D3 support this complex defense system? Which mechanisms are positively influenced by adequate Vitamin D3 supply? Research in recent years has uncovered surprising connections between Vitamin D3 status and the functionality of various immune cells. From strengthening innate immunity to modulating T and B cells, and regulating inflammatory processes – the effects of Vitamin D3 on the immune system are diverse and complex. Current studies show that an optimal Vitamin D3 level can not only reduce the risk of infection but also significantly contribute to the regulation of excessive immune reactions. The following sections illuminate the various mechanisms of this fascinating interaction between Vitamin D3 and our immune system.

„Epidemiological studies demonstrate a clear connection between vitamin D deficiency and increased susceptibility to infections, particularly respiratory diseases.“

3. 2. 1. Strengthening of Innate Immunity

The strengthening of innate immunity is a complex process influenced by various factors. Vitamin D plays a key role by directly interacting with immune cells and optimizing their functions [s175]. This interaction occurs through specific vitamin D receptors on immune cells, which, when vitamin D levels are sufficient, stimulate the production of important antimicrobial peptides such as cathelicidin and defensins. A particularly important aspect is the interaction between gut microbiota and the immune system [s176]. The gut flora produces essential B vitamins that are indispensable for immune homeostasis. To support these processes, a fiber-rich diet with fermented foods like sauerkraut or kefir is recommended. These promote a healthy gut flora and thereby indirectly support the immune system. Research shows that β-glucans can function as natural immune trainers [s177]. They essentially prepare the immune system for future infections, similar to preventive training. This can be practically achieved through the regular consumption of mushrooms such as shiitake or oyster mushrooms, which are rich in β-glucans. Vitamin C and zinc prove to be important partners in immune defense [s178]. Vitamin C enhances the activity of natural killer cells and supports lymphocyte proliferation. A zinc deficiency, on the other hand, can significantly impair the function of immune cells. A balanced diet rich in fresh fruits and vegetables, as well as high-quality animal products, can serve as a preventive measure. Particularly interesting is the local production of active vitamin D directly at infection sites [s179]. This occurs through the enzyme CYP27B1 in immune cells and leads to the formation of 1,25-dihydroxyvitamin D, which stimulates the expression of antimicrobial peptides. To support this mechanism, regular sun exposure of 15-20 minutes daily (considering skin type) is recommended. The activation of pattern recognition receptors (PRRs) on immune cells is another important mechanism of innate immunity [s180]. Plant-based immunomodulators can further stimulate this natural defense. This can be practically achieved through the consumption of immune-boosting herbs such as echinacea or ginger. Epidemiological studies demonstrate a clear correlation between vitamin D deficiency and increased susceptibility to infections [s181]. This is particularly evident in respiratory diseases. During the winter months, when natural vitamin D production from sunlight is limited, targeted supplementation may be advisable. The modulation of the immune response by vitamin D [s182] is also reflected in its ability to dampen excessive inflammatory reactions while promoting the production of protective anti-inflammatory cytokines. This is especially important in the prevention of autoimmune diseases and severe infection courses.

Practical recommendations for strengthening innate immunity include:
- Regular moderate exercise outdoors
- Sufficient sleep (7-9 hours)
- Stress reduction through relaxation techniques
- A balanced diet with plenty of whole grains, legumes, and colorful vegetables
- Regular consumption of fermented foods
- Adequate fluid intake (about 30-35 ml per kg of body weight)

These measures synergistically support the various mechanisms of innate immunity and contribute to a robust immune defense.

Glossary

Cathelicidin

An endogenous protein with antibiotic properties that can destroy the cell membranes of bacteria, viruses, and fungi.

Cytokines

Signaling molecules of the immune system that enable communication between different immune cells.

Immune Homeostasis

The balanced equilibrium of the immune system that oscillates between readiness for defense and tolerance.

Lymphocyte Proliferation

The proliferation of certain white blood cells in response to pathogens.

Pattern Recognition Receptors

Sensors of the immune system that can recognize typical structures of pathogens.

3. 2. 2. Impact on T-cells and B-cells

he effect of Vitamin D3 on T-cells and B-cells is a fascinating process that significantly contributes to the regulation of our immune system. Particularly noteworthy is the differentiated control of various immune cell types, which ensures a balanced immune response [s183]. An important aspect is the influence on regulatory T-cells (Tregs), whose numbers are increased by Vitamin D3. These Tregs act as natural "brakes" on the immune system, preventing excessive immune reactions [s184]. This is especially relevant in the prevention of autoimmune diseases. Individuals at increased risk for autoimmune diseases should therefore pay particular attention to their Vitamin D3 levels, for example, through regular outdoor activities during midday—naturally considering appropriate sun protection. Research also shows an interesting interaction between Vitamin D3 and IgA production in the small intestine [s183]. IgA is an important antibody that particularly protects mucous membranes. To support this protective effect, a gut-friendly diet with prebiotic foods such as chicory, Jerusalem artichokes, or artichokes is recommended. These promote a healthy gut flora and thereby indirectly support IgA production. Another significant effect of Vitamin D3 is the modulation of T-helper cells type 17 (Th17) [s184]. These cells play an important role in inflammatory processes, and their controlled activity is essential for a balanced immune response. In practice, this balancing effect can be supported by regular moderate exercise, as physical activity also contributes to the regulation of immune function. Particularly interesting is the role of Vitamin D3 during pregnancy [s184]. At the fetomaternal interface, it acts as a key regulator of immune function, ensuring a balanced relationship between infection defense and tolerance. Pregnant women should therefore regularly check their Vitamin D3 status and, if necessary, supplement after consulting their doctor. The lymphocyte count is positively influenced by Vitamin D3 supplementation, as studies show [s183]. This is particularly relevant during times of increased infection risk. To support this effect, a balanced diet rich in antioxidants, such as those found in colorful vegetables and berries, is recommended. The regulation of B-cell activity by Vitamin D3 is evident in controlled proliferation and differentiation [s184]. This is important for balanced antibody production. In practice, this function can be supported by sufficient and high-quality sleep, as important regeneration processes of the immune system occur during nighttime rest.

The complex interaction between Vitamin D3 and the adaptive immune system underscores the necessity of a holistic view of immune health. In addition to Vitamin D3 levels, factors such as stress management, adequate hydration, and a balanced work-life balance play an important role in an optimally functioning immune system.

Glossary

Immunoglobulin A

A Y-shaped protein that acts as the first line of defense on mucous membranes such as the nose, mouth, and intestines, trapping pathogens.

Lymphocyte

Small white blood cells specialized in recognizing and combating specific pathogens.

Regulatory T-cells

Special white blood cells that conduct and monitor other immune cells. They can stop harmful immune reactions.

3. 2. 3. Reduction of Infection Risk

he reduction of infection risk is based on a complex interplay of various factors, with adequate supply of essential <u>micronutrients</u> playing a central role [s185]. Especially during times of increased infection risk, optimal nutrient supply is of crucial importance. Studies show that individuals with a pronounced deficiency in certain micronutrients can reduce their infection risk by up to 44% through targeted supplementierung [s186]. This highlights the enormous preventive potential of optimized nutrient supply. To utilize this potential in daily life, a varied diet with a particular focus on nutrient-rich foods is recommended. Specifically, this means consuming at least five servings of differently colored fruits and vegetables daily, with each color representing different micronutrients. Research has shown that vitamins A, D, C, E, B6, and B12, as well as folate, zinc, iron, copper, and selenium, work <u>synergistically</u> to strengthen immune defense [s185]. A practical approach to optimizing supply is the development of a personal "immune protection meal plan." This should specifically combine nutrient-rich foods—such as pumpkin seeds for zinc, Brazil nuts for selenium, and citrus fruits for vitamin C. Particular attention should be paid to the role of omega-3 fatty acids in infection defense [s187]. These essential fatty acids support the resolution of inflammatory processes and thereby optimize the immune response. In practical terms, this means consuming fatty fish twice a week or, for a vegan diet, relying on high-quality algae oils. An innovative approach to infection prevention is the combination of vitamin D supplementation with targeted therapeutic measures [s188]. This can be particularly significant in the prevention of respiratory diseases. In daily life, this can be implemented through a combination of regular outdoor exercise—ideally 30-60 minutes daily—and need-based vitamin D supplementation. It is also important to consider individual risk factors. Certain population groups have an increased micronutrient requirement or inadequate intake [s185]. This includes, for example, older adults, pregnant women, or individuals with chronic illnesses. For these groups, targeted supplementation under medical supervision may be advisable. An often underestimated aspect of infection prevention is the importance of gut health. A balanced gut flora significantly supports immune function. Practically, this can be achieved through regular consumption of fermented foods such as kefir, kimchi, or sauerkraut, as well as the intake of <u>prebiotic</u> fibers. The implementation of these preventive measures should ideally occur year-round, with particular attention to vitamin D supply during the winter months. A practical approach is the development of a personal "immune protection routine," which includes not only nutrition but also adequate sleep, regular exercise, and stress management. The cost-effectiveness of micronutrient supplementation as a preventive measure [s187] makes it an attractive option for public health. However, supplementation should always be understood as a complement to a balanced diet, not as a substitute.

Glossary

Micronutrient
Essential substances such as vitamins, minerals, and trace elements that the body cannot produce itself and needs in small amounts.

Prebiotic
Indigestible food components that promote the growth and activity of beneficial gut bacteria.

Synergistic
The interaction of various factors, where the overall effect is greater than the sum of individual effects.

3. 2. 4. Modulation of the Inflammatory Response

he modulation of the inflammatory response by Vitamin D3 manifests as a complex and finely tuned process that encompasses various mechanisms. Particularly noteworthy is Vitamin D3's ability to specifically intervene in and regulate inflammatory processes [s189]. This occurs, among other things, through the reduction of pro-inflammatory signaling molecules such as TNF-α, while simultaneously activating anti-inflammatory mechanisms. A fascinating aspect is the newly discovered role of arginase activation as an anti-inflammatory mechanism [s189]. This insight opens new therapeutic perspectives, especially for skin diseases with an inflammatory component. In practice, this can be implemented, for example, through a combination of adequate Vitamin D3 supply and skin-friendly care. Individuals with skin issues should particularly pay attention to their Vitamin D3 levels and consider supplementation if necessary. In autoimmune diseases, a particularly interesting correlation emerges: low Vitamin D3 levels often correlate with increased disease activity [s190]. This is especially relevant for patients with conditions such as multiple sclerosis or rheumatoid arthritis. Practically, this means that affected individuals should regularly check their Vitamin D status and develop a personalized supplementation strategy in consultation with their physician. The genetic component of Vitamin D's effect, which is evident in polymorphisms of the Vitamin D receptor (VDR) [s190], underscores the necessity of a personalized approach. This also explains why individuals may respond differently to Vitamin D supplementation. A practical consequence is the recommendation to monitor individual Vitamin D supply through regular blood tests. Physical activity plays an important complementary role in modulating inflammatory responses [s191]. Regular moderate exercise reduces pro-inflammatory zytokine and promotes the production of anti-inflammatory signaling molecules. A practical approach is to integrate 30-45 minutes of moderate exercise daily, ideally outdoors, which additionally supports the body's own Vitamin D production. In the therapeutic application of Vitamin D3 for inflammation modulation, there are currently no uniform dosage recommendations [s192]. However, research suggests that higher doses under medical supervision may be beneficial for certain conditions. Regular monitoring of blood values and a gradual adjustment of dosage are important in this context.

A practical tip for everyday life is the combination of various inflammation-modulating strategies:
- Regular monitoring of Vitamin D levels
- Adjusted physical activity
- Anti-inflammatory diet rich in omega-3 fatty acids
- Stress reduction through relaxation techniques
- Sufficient sleep for immune system regeneration

This holistic approach can optimally support the inflammation-modulating effect of Vitamin D3 and contribute to improved health.

Glossary

Arginase
An enzyme that breaks down the amino acid arginine, thereby exerting anti-inflammatory effects.

Polymorphism
Naturally occurring variations in the DNA sequence that can lead to different expressions of a gene.

TNF-α
A signaling molecule of the immune system that is released during inflammation and can cause fever and tissue damage.

Summary - 3. 2. Immune System and Infection Defense

- Vitamin D3 interacts directly with immune cells through specific receptors and stimulates the production of antimicrobial peptides such as cathelicidin.
- The gut microbiota produces B vitamins, which are essential for immune homeostasis.
- β-glucans from mushrooms act as natural immune trainers, preparing the immune system for future infections.
- At infection sites, immune cells produce locally active vitamin D through the enzyme CYP27B1.
- Vitamin D3 increases the number of regulatory T cells (Tregs), which prevent excessive immune reactions.
- Vitamin D3 modulates type 17 helper T cells (Th17) for a balanced immune response.
- At the fetomaternal interface, vitamin D3 acts as a key regulator between infection defense and tolerance.
- Individuals with micronutrient deficiencies can reduce their infection risk by up to 44% through targeted supplementation.
- Vitamins A, D, C, E, B6, B12, as well as folate, zinc, iron, copper, and selenium work synergistically in immune defense.
- Polymorphisms of the vitamin D receptor (VDR) explain different individual responses to supplementation.
- Arginase activation has been identified as a new anti-inflammatory mechanism of vitamin D3.
- Low vitamin D3 levels correlate with increased disease activity in autoimmune diseases.

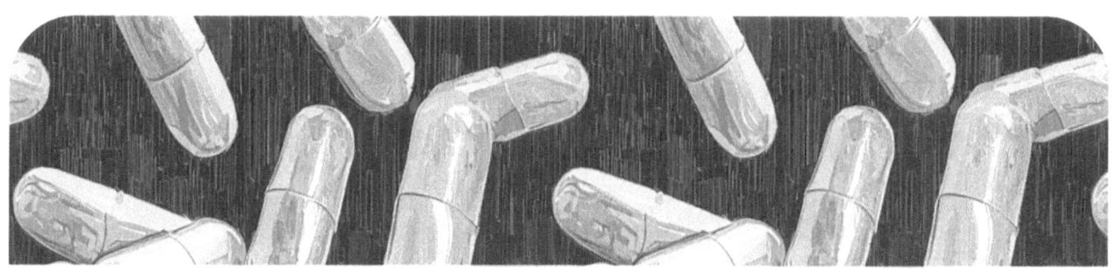

Review - 3. Effects and Benefits of Vitamin D3 Supplementation

- Vitamin D3 activates the production of antimicrobial peptides such as cathelicidin and defensins through specific vitamin D receptors on immune cells.
- The gut microbiota produces essential B vitamins for immune homeostasis and influences mineral absorption.
- β-glucans act as natural immune trainers, preparing the immune system for future infections.
- The local production of active vitamin D by the enzyme CYP27B1 occurs directly at infection sites.
- Regulatory T cells (Tregs) are increased by vitamin D3 and prevent excessive immune reactions.
- IgA production in the small intestine is modulated by vitamin D3, protecting mucous membranes.
- Vitamin D3 reduces pro-inflammatory signaling molecules such as TNF-α while simultaneously activating anti-inflammatory mechanisms.
- The activation of arginase has been discovered as a new anti-inflammatory mechanism of vitamin D3.
- Polymorphisms of the vitamin D receptor (VDR) explain different individual responses to supplementation.
- Individuals with vitamin D deficiency can reduce their infection risk by up to 44% through targeted supplementation.
- The highest bone density is achieved between the ages of 25 and 35.
- The body absorbs only 15-20% of the ingested calcium, with vitamin D3 optimizing this absorption.
- A daily intake of 800-1000 IU of vitamin D can reduce the risk of falls by 22%.
- The combined supplementation of calcium and vitamin D lowers the overall fracture risk by 15% and the risk of hip fractures by 30%.

- During pregnancy, vitamin D3 acts as a key regulator of immune function at the fetomaternal interface.

- But how can the optimal dosage be determined, and what safety aspects should be considered in supplementation?

4. Safety and Monitoring

he safe and controlled intake of Vitamin D3 raises questions for many people: How can one reliably determine their own Vitamin D status? What threshold values should be considered, and when might supplementation become dangerous? Monitoring Vitamin D supply requires a fundamental understanding of measurement methods and their interpretation. Not only pure laboratory values play a role—seasonal fluctuations and individual factors such as pre-existing conditions or medication use must also be taken into account. Particularly in the case of certain underlying conditions such as kidney insufficiency or sarcoidosis, Vitamin D3 supplementation requires careful monitoring. How can one find the right balance between adequate supply and potential overdose? The following chapters illuminate the various aspects of safely handling Vitamin D3 and highlight what should be particularly noted during regular monitoring. Only those who understand the essential fundamentals can make an informed decision about their own supplementation.

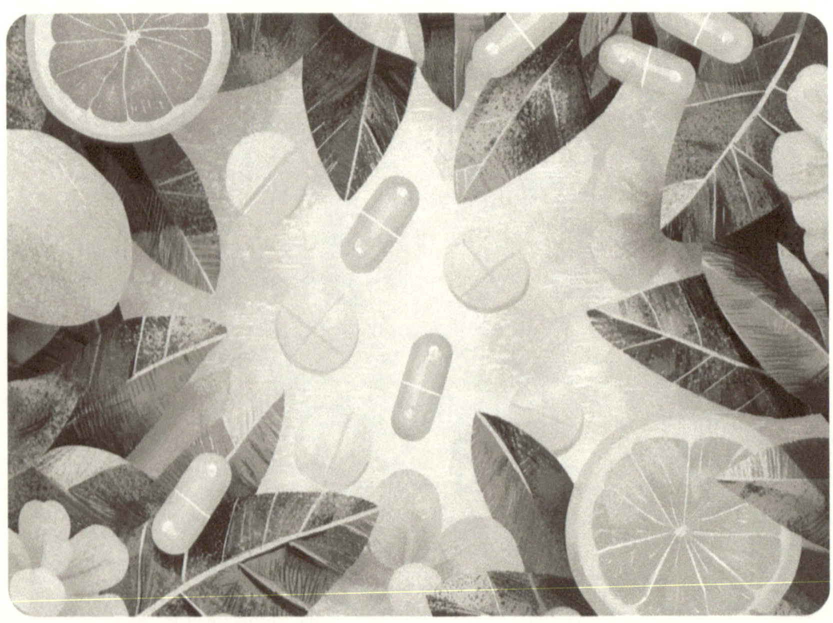

4. 1. Vitamin D Blood Levels

he determination of the vitamin D level in the blood is a central aspect for the safe and effective supplementation of vitamin D3. But how can the vitamin D status be reliably assessed? What methods are available, and what do the measured values actually mean? Particularly interesting is the question of optimal values—scientific discussion shows that defining a 'healthy' vitamin D level is more complex than initially assumed. Regular monitoring of vitamin D status not only allows for individual adjustment of supplementation but also provides important insights into overall health. The interpretation of the measurements requires consideration of various factors such as season, lifestyle, and personal health situation. A well-founded understanding of blood values and their significance is the key to safe and effective vitamin D supplementation.

„The LC-MS/MS method is considered the gold standard for determining vitamin D levels in the blood and is recommended by the national health and nutrition survey due to its improved sensitivity, accuracy, and reproducibility.“

4. 1. 1. Optimal Vitamin D Levels

The optimal vitamin D level in the blood is an important health indicator, determined by measuring 25hydroxyvitamin_d (25(OH)D) [s193]. For most individuals, a blood level of 50 nmol/L (20 ng/mL) or higher is considered sufficient for bone health and overall well-being [s194]. Many experts even recommend a target range between 40 and 60 ng/mL for optimal health [s195]. Vitamin D levels are categorized into different classifications: a severe deficiency is indicated by levels below 30 nmol/L (12 ng/mL) [s196], which can have dramatic health consequences. Levels between 30 and 50 nmol/L are considered insufficient, while levels above 125 nmol/L (50 ng/mL) are classified as too high and potentially toxic [s194]. To achieve and maintain an optimal vitamin D level, experts recommend various measures. The daily recommended intake varies depending on age and life situation: adults should consume about 600 IU daily, while individuals over 70 need approximately 800 IU [s197]. For infants, 400-1000 IU is recommended, for children and adolescents 600-1000 IU, and adults should take 1500-2000 IU daily [s195]. Regular monitoring of vitamin D levels is particularly important, ideally twice a year—once in spring and once in autumn [s195]. This allows for individual adjustments in supplementation. Individuals who spend little time outdoors or have darker skin should pay special attention to their vitamin D intake [s198]. In practice, this means that from late March to late September, most people can meet their vitamin D needs through sunlight exposure [s198]. A short walk at midday, exposing the face and arms to the sun, can already be beneficial. In the winter months, however, supplementation is often necessary [s198]. Interestingly, recent studies also show a correlation between vitamin D status and COVID-19: adequate supply may be associated with a milder course of the disease [s199]. A daily intake of 5000 IU of vitamin D3 over two weeks was able to shorten the recovery time from certain COVID-19 symptoms in patients with suboptimal vitamin D status [s199]. There are various approaches to supplementation: while some individuals take vitamin D daily, monthly doses or large loading doses can also be effective [s200]. The latter normalizes vitamin D levels particularly quickly, while monthly doses take 3-5 months to reach plateau levels [s200]. It is important to note that the optimal serum concentration of 25-hydroxyvitamin D is still under discussion, and there are differences in mineral metabolism among various ethnic groups [s201]. A too high vitamin D level (over 100 ng/mL) can be toxic due to secondary hyperkalzaemie [s201]. A deficiency in vitamin D can have serious consequences, ranging from bone deformities in children (rickets) to bone pain in adults (osteomalacia) [s198]. Therefore, it is crucial to know one's vitamin D status and optimize it through appropriate measures.

4. 1. 2. Methods for Determining Vitamin D Status

The determination of vitamin D status is primarily conducted through blood tests, with various methods available. The most important and commonly used measurement is 25-hydroxyvitamin D (25(OH)D) in the blood [s202]. For the examination, a blood sample of approximately 6 ml is taken from a vein in the arm [s203]. Patients should inform their doctor about all medications and supplements taken before the blood draw; however, no special preparations are required [s204].

The analytical methods for determining vitamin D have significantly advanced in recent years. The most common techniques include:
- Chemiluminescence-Immunoassays (CLIA)
- Radioimmunoassay (RIA)
- High-Performance Liquid Chromatography (HPLC)
- Liquid Chromatography-Tandem-Mass Spectrometry (LC-MS/MS)
- ELISA technique [s205] [s202]

The LC-MS/MS method is considered the gold standard and is recommended by the national health and nutrition survey. It is characterized by improved sensitivity, accuracy, and reproducibility [s205]. This is particularly important, as variability between different testing methods can complicate the interpretation of results [s202]. Another interesting aspect is the measurement of vitamin D binding protein (VDBP) and the calculation of bioavailable vitamin D. A study involving various patient groups showed that VDBP levels were significantly lower in intensive care patients and higher in pregnant women compared to healthy controls [s206]. These additional parameters can provide valuable information about vitamin D metabolism but are not yet routinely established in clinical practice [s207]. For specific diagnostic questions, measuring 1,25-dihydroxyvitamin D may also be useful. However, this test is not recommended for routine screening, as this metabolite has a very short half-life in the blood [s202]. It is primarily used in monitoring kidney issues or clarifying abnormal blood values [s204]. Practical recommendations for patients: 1. Ideally, have your vitamin D status checked twice a year, preferably in spring and autumn. 2. Keep an accurate list of your medications and supplements before the blood draw. 3. Inquire about the measurement method used and request a detailed explanation of the results. 4. Consider individual factors such as skin type, lifestyle, and season when interpreting the values. Research is continuously working on improving testing methods. Current developments aim to enhance the standardization of 25(OH)D measurement to ensure better comparability of results between different laboratories [s207]. New approaches, such as the simultaneous measurement of 25(OH)D and 24,25(OH)2D, could provide additional insights into vitamin D metabolism in the future [s207]. The use of modern analytical methods to predict vitamin D deficiency is also interesting. Studies have shown that multivariate logistic regression, neural networks, and decision tree analyses can be used to assess risk factors such as race, gender, season, and serum albumin levels [s208]. These models could help identify risk groups earlier and target treatment more effectively in the future.

Glossary

Chemiluminescence
A physical process in which chemical reactions lead to the emission
of light without producing heat.

ELISA
A laboratory technique for detecting proteins based on an enzymatic
color reaction, allowing for very precise measurements.

High-Performance Liquid Chromatography
A modern separation technique in which substances are pressed
through a column under high pressure to separate them from one
another.

Immunoassay
A laboratory method for detecting substances based on the specific
binding between antibodies and the molecules to be measured.

Mass Spectrometry
An analytical method for determining the mass of molecules
through ionization and subsequent measurement of their mass-to-
charge ratio.

Radioimmunoassay
A highly sensitive detection method that uses radioactively labeled
molecules to measure specific substances in the blood.

4. 1. 3. Interpretation of Test Results

The interpretation of vitamin D test results requires a nuanced understanding of various factors and thresholds. Laboratory reports present values either as "total vitamin D" or separately as vitamin D2 and D3. For clinical assessment, the sum of both values is relevant, as both forms exert similar effects in the body [s209]. The definition of thresholds is handled somewhat differently in the professional community. While some authorities define insufficiency at values between 12 and 19 ng/mL and deficiency at less than 12 ng/mL [s210], others consider values below 50 nmol/L (20 ng/mL) as deficient [s211]. These differing definitions can be confusing for patients. A practical tip: Ask your doctor to explain the thresholds used and document them along with your measurements. When interpreting the results, various influencing factors must be considered. Low values can have multiple causes: insufficient intake through food or sunlight, absorption disorders, or issues with conversion to the active form [s209]. A practical example: A patient with chronic inflammatory bowel disease may exhibit low values despite adequate sunlight exposure and supplementation, as absorption in the intestine is impaired. Interestingly, most people with vitamin D deficiency initially show no obvious symptoms [s212]. However, over the long term, there may be a drop in calcium levels and a secondary hyperfunction of the parathyroid glands. This underscores the importance of regular monitoring, especially in at-risk groups. The praevalenz of vitamin D deficiency is remarkably high worldwide, with significant differences among various population and age groups [s211]. A substantial percentage of individuals have values below 20 ng/mL [s213]. These epidemiological data should be considered in the individual assessment of test results. Patients with specific underlying conditions require special attention. A vitamin D assessment is particularly important for individuals with malabsorptionssyndromen, kidney failure, or unexplained bone pain [s214]. In such cases, closer monitoring of values is advisable. Caution is warranted when interpreting high values. Toxic vitamin D levels typically arise from excessive supplementation [s209]. A practical piece of advice: Keep a supplementation diary and regularly discuss the dosage with your doctor. If toxic levels are reached, supplementation must be stopped immediately to prevent organ damage. The standardization of testing methods remains a challenge. The interassay variability complicates the development of uniform guidelines for assessing vitamin D status [s215]. A practical tip for patients: Have your follow-up tests conducted in the same laboratory whenever possible to ensure comparability of values. Routine monitoring after supplementation is only necessary in certain clinical conditions treated by a specialist [s214]. For most individuals, regular checks in spring and autumn are sufficient to optimize supply.

Glossary

Interassay Variability
Refers to fluctuations in measurement results between different test executions or laboratories, even when the same sample is tested.

4. 1. 4. Seasonal Fluctuations in Blood Values

he seasonal fluctuations of vitamin D blood levels follow a characteristic annual rhythm influenced by various environmental and behavioral factors. Studies show significant differences between the seasons, with average 25ohd levels of 45.8 ng/ml in winter and 55.24 ng/ml in summer [s216]. This natural fluctuation has far-reaching implications for various health aspects. Particularly interesting is the relationship between seasonal vitamin D fluctuations and other blood values. Significant seasonal differences in lipid profiles have been demonstrated, with cholesterol, LDL, and HDL values exhibiting seasonal variations. Interestingly, triglyceride levels remain largely unaffected by these fluctuations [s216]. These findings are especially relevant for the interpretation of blood tests—cholesterol levels in winter may need to be assessed differently than comparable levels in summer. Blood pressure also shows clear seasonal fluctuations, independent of vitamin D supplementation. The average reduction in systolic blood pressure from winter to summer is a notable -6.6 mm Hg [s217]. For patients with hypertension, this means they may need to adjust their medication seasonally—a decision that should, of course, be coordinated with their treating physician. A practical aspect concerns the prevention of winter-related health issues. Supplementation with vitamin D3 and calcium during the winter months can effectively counterbalance the natural seasonal changes in calciotropic hormones and bone markers [s218]. This is particularly important for individuals in northern latitudes, where winter UV radiation is insufficient for adequate endogenous vitamin D production. Interesting insights also come from animal studies, which show that the highest 25OHD levels are reached after grazing and during peak sunlight exposure [s219]. These observations can be translated to humans: those who spend regular time outdoors in summer can naturally replenish their vitamin D stores. The monthly distribution of vitamin D levels shows a significant irregularity in non-supplemented individuals, with the lowest values in March and peak values in August and September [s220]. Practically, this means that a vitamin D measurement in late winter can provide important clues regarding potential supplementation needs. These seasonal fluctuations are particularly relevant for individuals with chronic conditions. In patients with chronic obstructive pulmonary disease, a clear correlation between vitamin D levels and the frequency of respiratory infections has been observed [s221]. This finding underscores the importance of adequate vitamin D supply, especially during the winter months. A practical tip for managing seasonal fluctuations: keep a "vitamin D diary" in which you document your blood values, sunlight exposure, and supplementation. This helps identify individual patterns and adjust supply accordingly. Discuss the results with your doctor to develop an optimal strategy tailored to your personal situation.

Glossary

calciotropic hormones
Hormones that regulate calcium balance in the body, primarily parathyroid hormone and calcitonin. They control calcium absorption in the intestine and calcium deposition in the bones.

lipid profile
A compilation of various blood fat values used to assess metabolism and cardiovascular risk.

systolic blood pressure
The upper blood pressure value that occurs when the heart muscle contracts. It indicates the pressure in the arteries during the heart's ejection phase.

Summary - 4. 1. Vitamin D Blood Levels

- 25-Hydroxyvitamin D (25(OH)D) is the most important indicator of vitamin D status in the blood.
- A severe vitamin D deficiency is present at levels below 30 nmol/L (12 ng/mL).
- Many experts recommend an optimal target range between 40-60 ng/mL.
- The LC-MS/MS method is considered the gold standard for vitamin D determination.
- VDBP levels are significantly lower in intensive care patients and higher in pregnant women compared to healthy individuals.
- Multivariate regression models and neural networks are used to predict vitamin D deficiency.
- Interassay variability between different testing methods complicates uniform interpretation.
- Seasonal fluctuations show average values of 45.8 ng/mL in winter and 55.24 ng/mL in summer.
- Vitamin D levels correlate with seasonal changes in lipid profiles and blood pressure.
- The lowest vitamin D values typically occur in March, while the highest are seen in August/September.
- A daily intake of 5000 IU of vitamin D3 over two weeks can shorten recovery time in COVID-19 patients.
- Monthly vitamin D doses require 3-5 months to reach plateau levels.

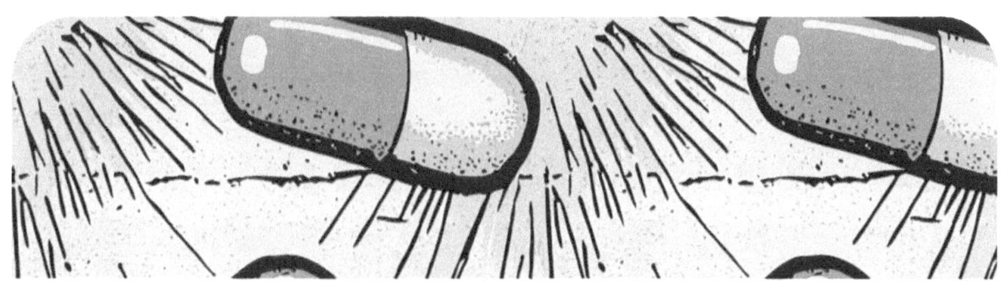

4. 2. Overdose and Toxicity

he question of the safe intake of Vitamin D3 concerns many people considering supplementation. At what dosage does this otherwise healthy vitamin become a risk? How can one recognize the first signs of an overdose? And what consequences can excessive intake have for the body? The line between therapeutic effect and potential toxicity is narrower for Vitamin D3 than often assumed. While moderate doses strengthen the immune system and promote bone health, excessive amounts can have serious health consequences. Particularly insidious: the symptoms of an overdose often develop gradually and can initially be easily overlooked. Therefore, a precise understanding of the safety limits and possible warning signs is essential for anyone supplementing with Vitamin D3. The following sections detail what to pay attention to when taking it.

„*A vitamin D overdose can manifest through a variety of symptoms that are often initially underestimated or misinterpreted and develop gradually.*"

4. 2. 1. Symptoms of Vitamin D Overdose

Vitamin D overdose can manifest through a variety of symptoms that are often initially underestimated or misinterpreted. The first signs are frequently nonspecific and develop gradually, making them easy to overlook [s222]. Affected individuals often report general weakness, persistent fatigue, and a reduced appetite. These symptoms can mistakenly be attributed to other causes, complicating early detection. A central mechanism of Vitamin D toxicity is the development of a hyperkalzaemie - that is, elevated calcium levels in the blood [s223]. This can have far-reaching consequences for various organ systems. In the digestive tract, symptoms such as nausea, vomiting, and persistent constipation may develop [s222]. A typical example from practice: a patient who independently took high doses of Vitamin D supplements for several months initially complained of recurring stomach pains and loss of appetite before further symptoms appeared. Particularly characteristic are also changes affecting kidney function. Affected individuals often notice increased thirst and a greater need to urinate [s222]. The urine may have a cloudy consistency [s224]. An important note for patients: If you notice that you are drinking significantly more than usual and need to go to the bathroom more frequently, you should have this checked by a doctor, especially if you are taking Vitamin D supplements. In advanced stages, neurological and psychological symptoms may also occur. These range from confusion and mood swings to severe conditions such as psychoses or even comatose states [s225]. The cardiovascular system can also be affected, which may manifest as arrhythmias or high blood pressure [s225]. Externally, various skin changes may appear: dry, cracked skin, increased sensitivity to light, and in some cases, even yellowish-orange discolored areas of skin [s224]. A practical tip: Pay particular attention to changes in the face, such as chapped lips or increased sensitivity to sunlight. Particularly dangerous is the fact that a Vitamin D overdose can weaken bones and lead to organ damage in the heart and kidneys [s223]. To avoid this, adherence to the recommended maximum amounts is essential: Adults should not consume more than 100 micrograms per day. For children between 1 and 10 years, the limit is 50 micrograms daily, and for infants under one year, a maximum of 25 micrograms [s223]. An important practical piece of advice: Keep a symptom diary if you are taking Vitamin D supplements. Note any abnormalities such as increased thirst, fatigue, or mood changes. This can help your doctor detect a possible overdose early. At the first signs of a potential overdose, medical advice should be sought immediately. Symptoms may worsen even after discontinuing Vitamin D, as it accumulates in fat tissue and is only slowly broken down. Regular monitoring of Vitamin D and calcium levels in the blood is advisable when taking Vitamin D supplements, especially with higher-dose products.

Glossary

Psychosis

A severe mental state in which individuals lose touch with reality. Characterized by delusions, hallucinations, or significantly altered behavior.

4. 2. 2. Risks of Hypercalcemia

hypercalcaemie, or elevated calcium levels in the blood, represents one of the most dangerous complications of vitamin D overdose. The risks associated with this metabolic disturbance are manifold and can have serious consequences for various organ systems [s226]. Particularly insidious is the fact that hypercalcemia can also occur with the intake of recommended vitamin D doses if there is individual hypersensitivity [s227]. The kidneys are often the first organ affected. In some patients, acute renal failure develops, which can be evidenced by elevated creatinine and urea levels in the blood [s228]. An example from clinical practice: A patient who took a high-dose vitamin D preparation for several months initially developed persistent vomiting. Only the laboratory examination revealed the underlying hypercalcemia and beginning kidney damage. Immediate treatment with fluid replacement, diuretics, and calcitonin could prevent more severe consequences [s228]. Children are particularly at risk, as accidental overdose can lead to hypercalcemia. Interestingly, a study showed that of 15 children with vitamin D overdose, only one developed manifest hypercalcemia [s229]. This may be related to the frequent vitamin D deficiency in the region, which possibly offers some protection. A frequently underestimated risk lies in the manufacturing and dosing of vitamin D preparations. A study found that 5% of patients had serum levels in the toxic range, with two cases being so severe that hospitalization was required [s230]. The median serum concentration in the overdose group was 185.5 ng/ml, which represents a significant exceedance of therapeutic limits [s230]. Practical recommendation for patients: Keep an accurate record of the vitamin D preparations taken and pay particular attention to the correct dosage. For magistral preparations, you should discuss the dosing instructions particularly carefully with the pharmacist. The diagnosis of hypercalcemia requires a comprehensive evaluation of the medical history and clinical symptoms [s226]. Typical laboratory findings, in addition to hypercalcemia, include elevated serum creatinine levels and high 25-OH vitamin D levels [s231]. Interestingly, liver values usually remain within the normal range, which can be helpful in differential diagnosis. A particular risk is posed by incorrect labeling of dietary supplements or excessively fortified foods [s231]. Patients should therefore only use preparations from trusted manufacturers and be cautious when combining various fortified products.

Recommendation for medical personnel: In patients with persistent vomiting and normal parathormon, vitamin D-induced hypercalcemia should always be considered [s228]. Early detection and treatment can prevent serious kidney damage. The prognosis of acute vitamin D toxicity with hypercalcemia is usually good with timely recognition and adequate treatment [s229]. Nevertheless, prevention through careful dosing and regular monitoring is the best way to minimize the risks of hypercalcemia.

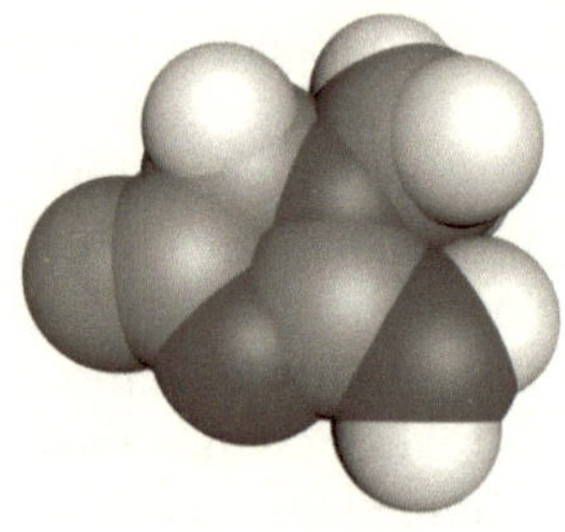

Creatinine [i12]

Glossary

Calcitonin
A hormone produced in the thyroid gland that lowers blood calcium levels by promoting the incorporation of calcium into bones.

Creatinine
A breakdown product of muscle metabolism that serves as an important marker for kidney function. Elevated levels indicate impaired kidney performance.

4. 2. 3. Safety Limits for Daily Intake

stablishing safe intake limits for Vitamin D3 is a complex issue, with various health organizations providing somewhat differing recommendations. The Endocrine Society sets the upper limit at 10,000 IU (International Units) daily, while other organizations recommend a more conservative approach of a maximum of 4,000 IU per day [s232]. These differing assessments highlight the ongoing scientific discussion regarding optimal safety limits. For practical application, it is important to understand that even the intake of 40 IU of Vitamin D3 increases the serum concentration of 25(OH)D by approximately 1 nM (0.4 ng/ml) [s233]. This allows for a better estimation of dosage: for instance, if a patient wishes to raise their Vitamin D level by 20 ng/ml, a theoretical dose of about 2,000 IU daily would be required. However, such calculations should always be conducted under medical supervision, as individual factors can significantly influence absorption and utilization. The tolerable upper intake level (UL) refers to the maximum chronic intake at which health risks are considered unlikely [s234]. A practical example: a person taking a Vitamin D supplement of 2,000 IU daily and additionally consuming vitamin D-fortified foods should keep track of and document their total intake. Particular caution is warranted with long-term supplementation. Studies indicate that doses exceeding 800 IU daily may be associated with an increased risk of hypercalcemia and hypercalciuria [s235]. A practical tip for supplementation: maintain a record of your intake and also note the consumption of vitamin D-rich or fortified foods. Different safety limits apply to various age groups. Children aged 9 and older, adolescents, and adults should not exceed 2,500 IU (62.5 μg) daily [s236]. Lower limits apply to younger children, which is particularly important to consider when using vitamin D supplements in families. Interestingly, research findings suggest that sun-deprived adults may require higher doses to maintain an optimal Vitamin D level (>75 nM or 30 ng/ml) [s233]. This underscores the importance of individualized dosing, taking into account factors such as sun exposure, skin type, and lifestyle. An important practical note for supplementation: choose the dosage according to your individual situation and have your Vitamin D levels checked regularly. Especially in the first weeks of supplementation, be vigilant for potential side effects and document them. The therapeutic range of Vitamin D3 may be narrower than previously assumed [s235]. Therefore, a cautious approach to high-dose preparations is advisable. A practical strategy is the "start low, go slow" principle: begin with a lower dose and only increase it as needed and under medical supervision.

For safe supplementation, the following recommendations can be summarized:
- Document your total daily intake from all sources
- Consider your individual situation (sun exposure, pre-existing conditions)
- Have your Vitamin D and calcium levels checked regularly
- Choose high-quality supplements from reputable manufacturers
- Always discuss dosage changes with your doctor

4. 2. 4. Treatment of Vitamin D Intoxication

The treatment of vitamin D intoxication requires a swift and systematic approach, as the consequences can be severe. The first and most important measure is to immediately stop vitamin D intake [s237]. This applies to both supplements and fortified foods. A central aspect of treatment is adequate fluid intake. Patients should drink large amounts of water to support kidney function and promote the excretion of excess substances [s237]. Clinical practice has shown that especially at the first signs of intoxication, increased fluid intake of 2-3 liters daily can be beneficial. Medical treatment primarily focuses on normalizing elevated calcium levels and supportive measures [s238]. In the hospital, extensive diagnostic tests are initially conducted, including blood and urine tests as well as imaging procedures [s239]. A typical treatment protocol may look as follows: 1. Intravenous fluid administration for rehydration 2. Monitoring of vital signs 3. Regular electrolyte checks 4. Administration of medications to lower calcium levels if necessary In cases of severe toxicity with hypercalcemia (serum calcium >14 mg/dL), specific medications are employed [s238]. In particularly severe cases, hemodialysis may become necessary, especially if kidney failure is imminent or if hyperkalzaemie does not respond adequately to medical therapy [s238]. The recovery time varies significantly among individuals. While mild cases often normalize within a few weeks, severe intoxications may require up to 6 months of treatment [s237]. A practical tip for those affected: Keep a symptom diary during the recovery phase and document your daily fluid intake.

Preventing long-term consequences is particularly important. Treatment must continue until blood values return to normal, as otherwise, there is a risk of permanent damage. Possible long-term complications include:
- Kidney and blood vessel damage
- Bone demineralization
- Chronic gastrointestinal issues
- Persistent muscle weakness [s237]

An interesting aspect is that toxicity can arise not only from excessive external intake but also from endogenous factors such as granulomatous diseases or certain lymphomas [s240]. This underscores the importance of thorough diagnostic evaluation.

For relatives and first responders, it is crucial to have relevant information available in emergencies:
- Age and weight of the affected person
- Type and amount of vitamin D preparation taken
- Time of last intake
- Existing preconditions [s239]

The prognosis is usually good with timely treatment; however, delayed interventions can lead to irreversible damage. A practical piece of advice for the period following acute treatment: Regularly monitor your kidney function and calcium levels, and initially avoid intense sun exposure [s241]. For aftercare, a structured plan is recommended: 1. Regular laboratory checks 2. Dietary adjustments 3. Gradual increase in physical activity 4. Close medical supervision In case of uncertainties regarding further vitamin D supplementation, medical advice should be sought [s241]. Individual dosing must be evaluated particularly carefully after intoxication.

Summary - 4. 2. Overdose and Toxicity

- Vitamin D overdose can manifest as hypercalcemia and psychoses. The median serum concentration in the overdose group was 185.5 ng/ml. Of 15 children with vitamin D overdose, only one developed manifest hypercalcemia. Serum levels in the toxic range were detected in 5% of patients. The intake of 40 IU of vitamin D3 increases the serum concentration of 25(OH)D by approximately 1 nM. Doses exceeding 800 IU daily may be associated with an increased risk of hypercalcemia. The Endocrine Society sets the upper limit at 10,000 IU daily. Children aged 9 and older should not exceed an intake of 2,500 IU daily. Severe intoxications may require up to 6 months of treatment. Toxicity can also arise from endogenous factors such as granulomatous diseases. Liver values usually remain within the normal range in vitamin D overdose. Acute renal insufficiency is indicated by elevated creatinine and urea levels.

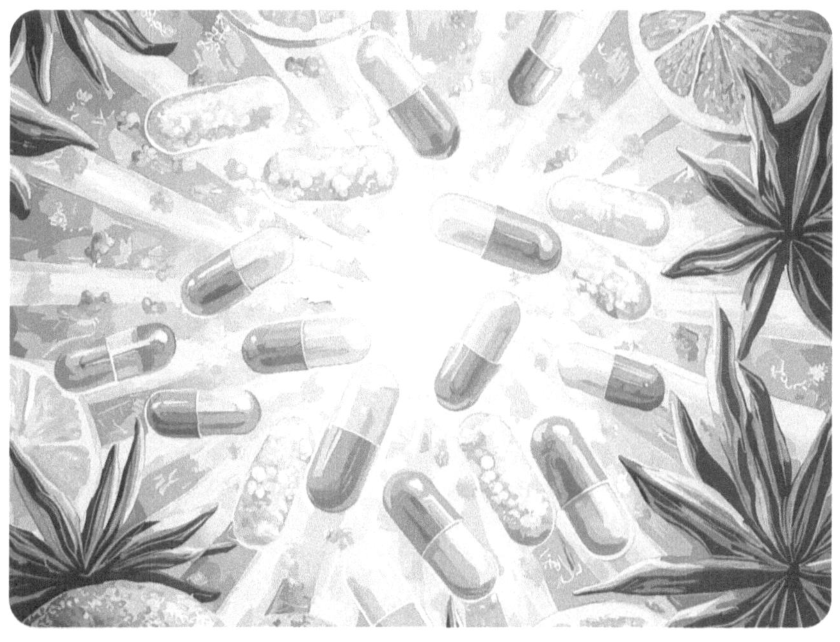

4. 3. Contraindications and Precautions

upplementation with vitamin D3 requires special attention and specific precautions in certain health situations. But which diseases and medications can influence vitamin D absorption and metabolism? How can the risk of overdose be minimized in the presence of underlying conditions? While the positive effects of adequate vitamin D supply are well documented, certain pre-existing conditions or medications can disrupt the delicate balance of vitamin D levels. A differentiated approach is particularly necessary in cases of kidney disease, sarcoidosis, hyperparathyroidism, or the use of anticonvulsants. The following sections illuminate the key contraindications and necessary precautions for vitamin D3 supplementation—essential knowledge for safe and effective use.

„*In patients with kidney diseases, the safe upper limit for daily vitamin D intake is 10,000 IU.*"

4. 3. 1. Vitamin D in Kidney Diseases

n patients with kidney diseases, vitamin D supplementation requires special attention and careful monitoring, as the kidneys play a central role in vitamin D metabolism. Treatment must be individually tailored to avoid both deficiency and overdose [s242]. It is important for affected individuals to know that supplementation should only begin after a thorough laboratory examination. In particular, the parathormon (PTH) level should be checked. If this is above the target range, a measurement of the 25(OH)D level should be performed [s243]. A practical example: In a chronic kidney patient with elevated PTH and a 25(OH)D level below 30 ng/mL, an ergocalciferol supplementation would typically be initiated. The safe upper limit for daily vitamin D intake in kidney diseases is 10,000 IU [s242]. This upper limit should never be exceeded, as it can lead to serious complications. Patients should keep a medication diary and regularly have their laboratory values checked.

Particular caution is warranted, as vitamin D overdose can lead to toxic effects more quickly in patients with kidney diseases than in healthy individuals. Symptoms of intoxication can be varied and include:
- Increased thirst and frequent urination (polyuria)
- Loss of appetite and nausea
- Constipation
- Fatigue
- Muscle cramps
- Bone pain [s242]

For treating physicians, it is crucial to closely monitor calcium and phosphate levels. Supplementation should be stopped if the corrected calcium level exceeds 10.2 mg/dL or the phosphate level exceeds 4.6 mg/dL [s243]. A practical tip for patients: Have your doctor write down your individual threshold values and document these along with your laboratory results.

The use of active vitamin D and its analogs in chronic kidney disease requires special attention, as these can lead to unwanted effects such as elevated calcium levels in the blood and adynamic bone disease [s244]. Patients should therefore be alert to the following warning signs and discuss them promptly with their doctor:
- Unusual fatigue
- Newly occurring bone pain
- Digestive problems
- Changes in urination

In severe cases, vitamin D intoxication can lead to kidney dysfunction, calcifications in the kidneys (nephrocalcinosis), and neurological symptoms such as consciousness disturbances or even seizures [s242]. Therefore, it is essential for patients to adhere to the prescribed dosage and attend regular check-ups. The research on vitamin D supplementation in chronic kidney disease shows varying results [s244]. While certain forms of vitamin D can reliably lower parathyroid hormone levels, the increase in fgf23 levels (Fibroblast Growth Factor 23) must be carefully monitored. Patients should therefore work closely with their nephrologist and regularly review the treatment regimen. A practical approach for therapy monitoring is to keep a health diary, in which, in addition to vitamin D intake, possible symptoms and general well-being are documented. This helps the treating physician to optimally adjust the therapy and recognize potential side effects early.

4. 3. 2. Caution with Sarcoidosis and Granulomatosis

n the case of <u>sarcoidosis</u> and other granulomatoesen diseases, special caution is required regarding vitamin D supplementation, as these conditions can significantly affect vitamin D metabolism. The reason lies in the unique metabolic situation: the granulomas that form in these diseases produce the enzyme 1α-hydroxylase [s245] in increased amounts. This leads to an enhanced conversion of vitamin D into its active form, which in turn increases the risk of hyperkalzaemie (elevated calcium levels in the blood). For affected individuals, it is essential to undergo a thorough baseline examination of calcium levels before starting vitamin D supplementation [s246]. This initial examination serves as an important starting point for the ongoing monitoring of calcium metabolism. A practical example: a patient with newly diagnosed sarcoidosis should first have their calcium and vitamin D levels determined before beginning supplementation. These values should be documented in a personal health diary. Interestingly, research findings indicate a complex relationship between vitamin D levels and disease activity in sarcoidosis. A low vitamin D level (<u>hypovitaminosis</u> D) appears to be associated with higher disease activity [s245]. This presents a particular challenge for doctors and patients: on one hand, vitamin D supplementation could potentially be beneficial, while on the other hand, there is a risk of hypercalcemia. For practical implementation, the following approach is recommended: 1. Regular monitoring of calcium levels, ideally every 3-4 weeks at the beginning of supplementation.

2. Keeping a detailed symptom diary with special attention to:

- Nausea

- Loss of appetite

- Increased fatigue

- Muscle or joint pain
- Increased thirst

A study involving 104 sarcoidosis patients showed that about 5% of patients developed hypercalcemia under calcium and vitamin D supplementation [s245]. However, it is important to note that supplementation was not the primary cause of hypercalcemia. This underscores the necessity of an individualized assessment of each case. In practice, this means that patients with sarcoidosis or other granulomatous diseases should closely coordinate their vitamin D supplementation with their treating physician. A sensible approach is the gradual introduction of supplementation with regular monitoring of relevant laboratory values.

Affected individuals should also learn to pay attention to early warning signs of hypercalcemia. These can be subtle and are often overlooked. A practical tip is to use a symptom checklist that is reviewed daily. Even seemingly harmless changes such as:
- Mild concentration difficulties
- Increased urination
- Digestive changes
- Unusual fatigue

should be documented and discussed with the treating physician. The dosage of vitamin D supplementation in these conditions should generally be set lower than in healthy individuals. Close monitoring and, if necessary, adjustment of the dose is essential for safe supplementation.

Glossary

Hypovitaminosis
A state of vitamin deficiency that falls below the recommended minimum level and can cause various health problems.

Sarcoidosis
An inflammatory systemic disease characterized by the formation of small nodules (granulomas) in various organs, most commonly in the lungs and lymph nodes.

4. 3. 3. Special Caution with Hyperparathyroidism

In the case of primary hyperparathyreoidismus (pHPT), utmost caution is required during vitamin D3 supplementation, as this condition already leads to a disturbed calcium metabolism [s247]. The excessive production of parathyroid hormone by the parathyroid glands can, in combination with vitamin D3, lead to a dangerous exacerbation of hyperkalzaemie. For affected individuals, a structured monitoring program is essential. Treatment must only occur under medical supervision [s248]. A specific example of the monitoring plan: In the first week after the start of therapy, the first check of biochemical parameters takes place, with further checks occurring in weeks 4, 8, and 12. In particular, calcium levels and kidney function are monitored.

Patients should maintain a detailed health diary, documenting the following aspects daily:
- General well-being
- Occurrence of fatigue or weakness
- Digestive issues
- Changes in urination
- Muscle or joint complaints

The situation is particularly critical for patients with additional hypercalciuria or urolithiasis (kidney stones). Here, the treating physician must carefully weigh the risks and benefits [s247]. A practical tip for affected individuals: In addition to the health diary, maintain a fluid intake log and ensure adequate hydration of at least 2.5 liters daily. In cases of suspected masked pHPT—meaning that the typical laboratory value changes are obscured by a concurrent vitamin D deficiency—special attention is required [s248]. In such cases, an initially unremarkable vitamin D3 supplementation can lead to a sudden unmasking of pHPT. Patients should therefore be trained to notice and document even subtle changes. An important exclusion: Patients with advanced renal insufficiency (estimated GFR below 30 ml/min/1.73 m²) require a specially tailored treatment protocol [s248]. Separate guidelines apply to this patient group, which must be coordinated with a nephrologist. For practical implementation, the following approach is recommended: 1. Create an individual monitoring plan together with your doctor 2. Maintain a laboratory value diary 3.

Document all medication intakes 4. Note any abnormalities or complaints 5. Schedule regular follow-up appointments

At the first signs of deterioration such as:
- Increased thirst
- More frequent urination
- Digestive disturbances
- Concentration difficulties

immediate contact with the treating physician should be made. Therapy monitoring should not only consider laboratory values but also the patient's subjective well-being. A holistic treatment approach that includes lifestyle factors such as diet and exercise has proven effective in practice.

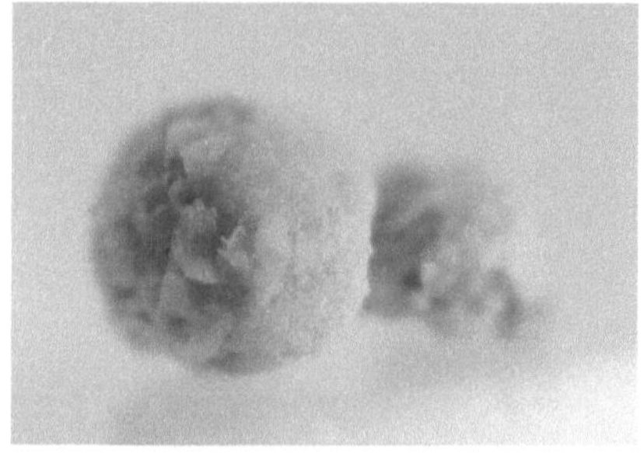

Urolithiasis [i13]

Glossary

Hypercalciuria
An increased calcium excretion in the urine that significantly raises the risk of kidney stones and can impair kidney function.

Nephrologist
A specialist in kidney diseases who focuses on the diagnosis and treatment of urinary system disorders.

Urolithiasis
The medical term for the formation of stones in the urinary system, which can lead to severe pain and kidney damage.

4. 3. 4. Adjustment when taking anticonvulsants

hen taking <u>anticonvulsants</u> (antiepileptics), special attention to vitamin D levels is required, as these medications can significantly affect vitamin D metabolism [s249]. This effect is particularly pronounced with the use of <u>carbamazepine</u>, which has been shown to reduce 25-hydroxy vitamin D levels (25OHD) [s249]. The underlying mechanism is based on the activation of the enzyme CYP3A4 in the liver by certain antiepileptics. This enzyme accelerates the breakdown of vitamin D into inactive <u>metabolites</u> [s250]. As a result of this increased metabolism, vitamin D levels in the body can drop significantly, which may have long-term negative effects on bone health [s250]. For patients who are on anticonvulsants long-term, this leads to important practical consequences:

1. Regular monitoring of vitamin D levels:
- A baseline measurement should be taken at the start of therapy
- Quarterly checks in the first year
- Subsequently, semi-annual reviews if values are stable

2. Adjustment of vitamin D supplementation:
- Higher dosages may be necessary
- Individual adjustments based on regular measurements
- Documentation of intake and measurement values in a therapy diary

A practical example illustrates the necessity of close monitoring: A patient who has been taking carbamazepine for two years should have their vitamin D levels checked every 6 months. If a vitamin D deficiency is detected, a higher supplementation dose may be necessary, which must be carefully <u>titrated</u>.

It is particularly important to pay attention to possible warning signs that may indicate a vitamin D deficiency:
- Increasing fatigue
- Muscle pain or weakness
- Increased susceptibility to infections
- Mood swings

For practical implementation, the following approach is recommended: 1. Keep a record of anticonvulsant and vitamin D intake 2. Document any symptoms that arise 3. Adhere to regular check-up appointments 4. Discuss any abnormalities promptly with the treating physician Research shows that long-term users of antiepileptics have not only lower vitamin D levels compared to control groups but also reduced bone density [s250]. This underscores the importance of proactive monitoring and supplementation. For treating physicians, it is important to know that the use of CYP3A4-inducing medications must be considered a potential risk factor for vitamin D deficiency [s251]. However, current studies also indicate that the influence of anticonvulsants on vitamin D status in certain patient groups has not yet been sufficiently investigated [s251]. This makes individual assessment and adjustment of therapy all the more important.

Another practical tip for those affected is to create a personal vitamin D management plan in collaboration with the treating physician. This should include the following aspects:
- Individually adjusted supplementation dose
- Schedule for follow-up examinations
- List of relevant symptoms for self-monitoring
- Emergency contacts for acute issues

Regular review and adjustment of this plan is essential for successful long-term therapy.

Anticonvulsants

Medications used to treat epileptic seizures that regulate electrical activity in the brain. Also known as antiepileptics.

Carbamazepine

A commonly prescribed anticonvulsant that is also used for nerve pain and bipolar disorder.

Metabolite

Intermediate and end products that arise during the conversion of substances in the body.

Titration

Gradual adjustment of a medication dose to achieve optimal effect with minimal side effects.

Summary - 4. 3. Contraindications and Precautions

- In cases of kidney disease, the safe upper limit for daily vitamin D intake is 10,000 IU. Supplementation should be discontinued if the corrected calcium level exceeds 10.2 mg/dL or the phosphate level exceeds 4.6 mg/dL. In sarcoidosis, granulomas produce the enzyme 1α-hydroxylase in increased amounts, leading to enhanced conversion of vitamin D into its active form. A study involving 104 sarcoidosis patients showed that approximately 5% developed hypercalcemia under calcium and vitamin D supplementation. In primary hyperparathyroidism, vitamin D3 supplementation can dangerously exacerbate hypercalcemia. A masked primary hyperparathyroidism may be obscured by a concurrent vitamin D deficiency. Carbamazepine has been shown to reduce 25-hydroxy vitamin D levels by activating the enzyme CYP3A4. Long-term users of antiepileptics not only exhibit lower vitamin D levels compared to control groups but also show reduced bone density.

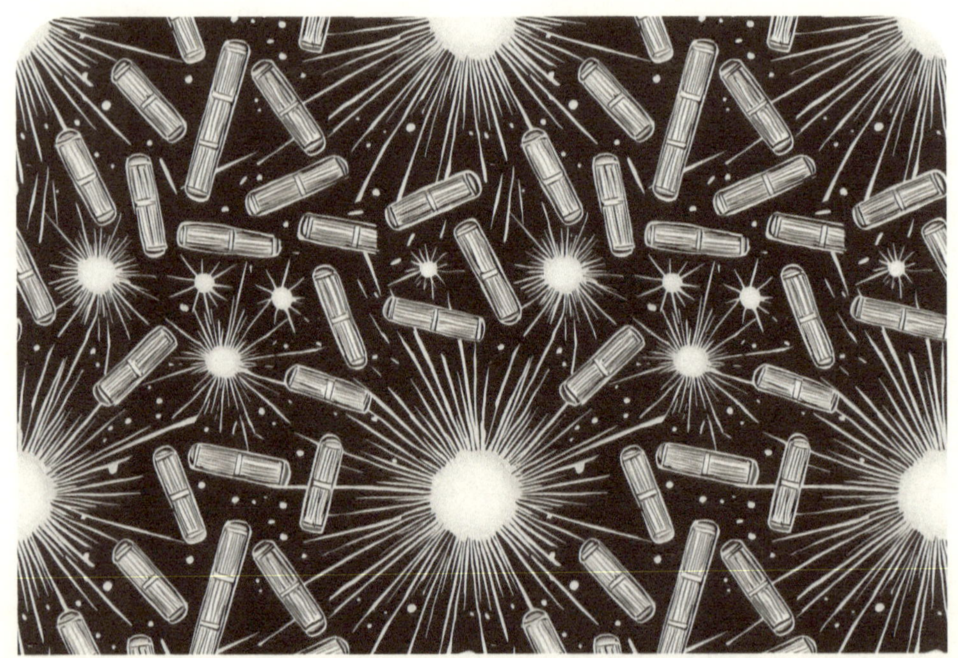

Review - 4. Safety and Monitoring

- The optimal vitamin D level is between 50-125 nmol/L, measured as 25-hydroxyvitamin D.
- A severe deficiency below 30 nmol/L can have dramatic health consequences.
- The LC-MS/MS method is considered the gold standard for vitamin D determination.
- Vitamin D-binding protein is significantly lower in intensive care patients and higher in pregnant women.
- The first signs of an overdose often develop gradually and can be easily overlooked.
- Vitamin D toxicity can weaken bones and lead to organ damage in the heart and kidneys.
- In sarcoidosis, granulomas produce the enzyme 1α-hydroxylase in increased amounts.
- About 5% of sarcoidosis patients develop hypercalcemia under supplementation.
- In primary hyperparathyroidism, vitamin D3 can dangerously exacerbate hypercalcemia.
- Anticonvulsants activate the enzyme CYP3A4, which accelerates the breakdown of vitamin D.
- As little as 40 IU of vitamin D3 increases serum concentration by approximately 1 nM.
- The tolerable upper intake level is 2,500 IU daily for children aged 9 and older and adults.
- Multivariate regression models can predict risk factors for vitamin D deficiency.

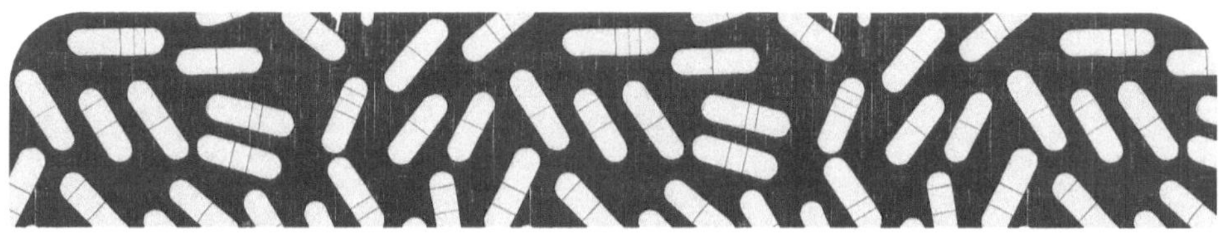

Free Additional Offers Planned

We are pleased to offer you free supplementary materials for this book in the future:

- An exclusive bonus chapter with additional content
- A compact summary of the entire book in PDF format

These materials are expected to be released in January 2025.
Feel free to visit our website today. Once our newsletter service launches (expected January 2025), you can register there for updates and won't miss any news about the free additional offers.

SaageBooks.com/vitamin_d3_supplementation-bonus-W81RER

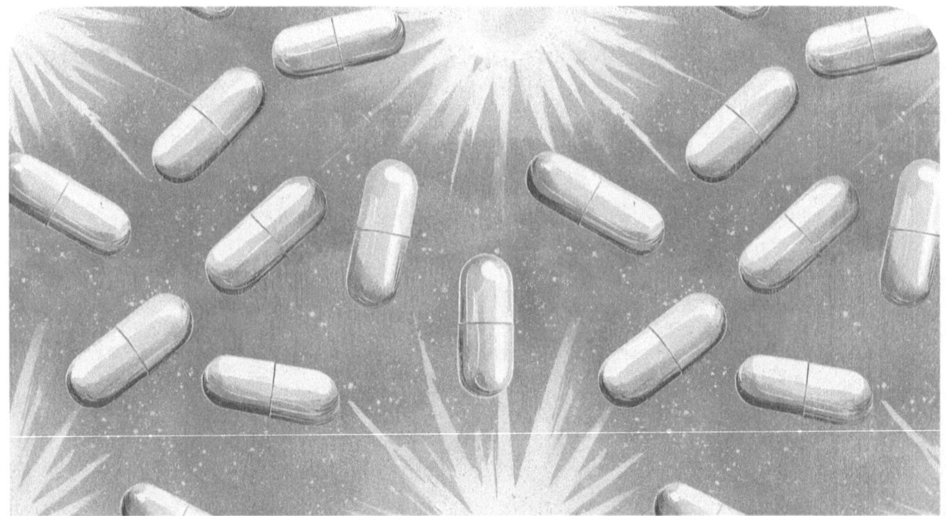

Dear readers,

I am deeply honored that you have taken the time to read my book from beginning to end. As an author, my greatest wish is to provide you with valuable insights and practical guidance. Your trust in my work means a lot to me. I hope the reading was enriching for you. If you have any questions or suggestions, please feel free to contact me through our website.

If you enjoyed this book, I would greatly appreciate an honest review. Your opinion matters to me and helps other readers make their decision. You can easily leave your honest rating on the sales platform where you purchased the book.
Thank you for your support!

Artemis Saage

Saage Media GmbH

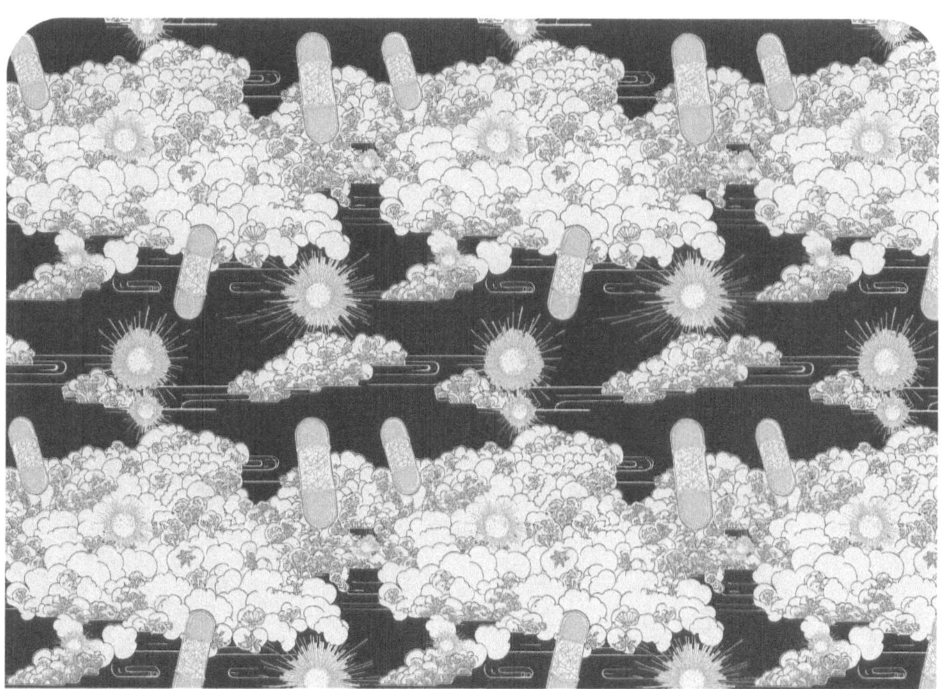

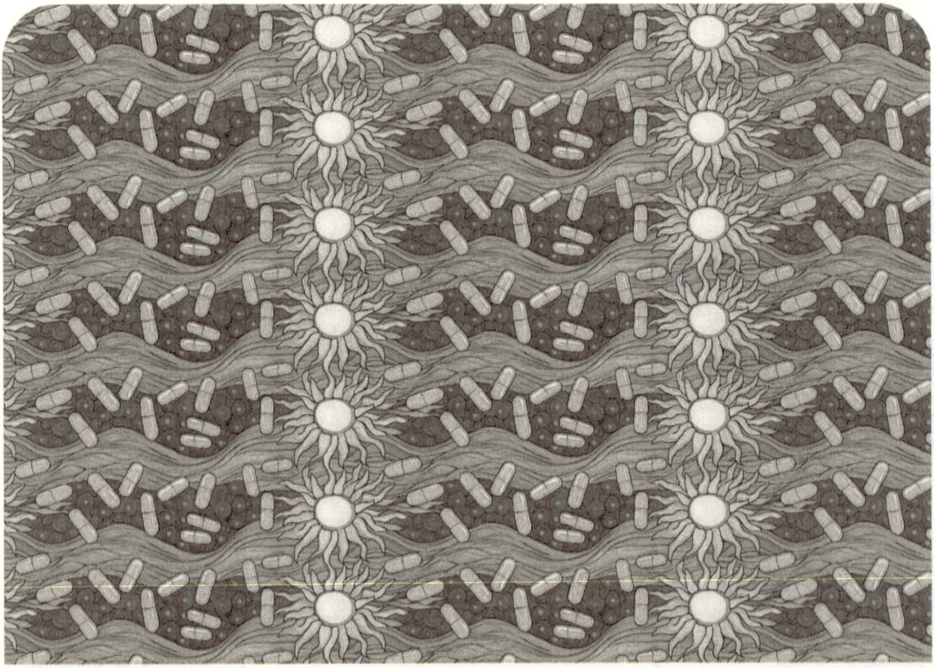

Sources

My sincere thanks go to all authors of the cited scientific and non-scientific sources, the operators of the referenced websites, and the creators of the images, graphics, and studies used, whose valuable work has significantly contributed to the creation of this book.
For more information, I recommend visiting the linked source websites.

All sources were last accessed on: 2024-12-20

[s1] - https://pubmed.ncbi.nlm.nih.gov/2825606/
Author: M F Holick, E Smith, S Pincus — **Title:** Skin as the site of vitamin D synthesis and target tissue for 1,25-dihydroxyvitamin D3. Use of calcitriol (1,25-dihydroxyvitamin D3) for treatment of psoriasis
by: US Department of AgricultureHuman Nutrition Research Center, Tufts University — **Release Date:** 1987-12
Website: PubMed — **Publisher:** Archives of Dermatology

[s2] - https://ec.europa.eu/health/scientific_committees/scheer/docs/sunbeds_co99a_en.pdf
Author: Michael F Holick, Tai C Chen, Zhiren Lu, Edward Sauter — **Title:** Vitamin D and Skin Physiology: A D-Lightful Story
Release Date: 2007 — **Website:** European Commission
Publisher: American Society for Bone and Mineral Research

[s3] - https://pubmed.ncbi.nlm.nih.gov/2839537/
Author: A R Webb, L Kline, M F Holick — **Title:** Influence of season and latitude on the cutaneous synthesis of vitamin D3: exposure to winter sunlight in Boston and Edmonton will not promote vitamin D3 synthesis in human skin
by: Boston University Medical School — **Release Date:** 1988-08
Website: PubMed — **Publisher:** J Clin Endocrinol Metab

[s4] - https://lpi.oregonstate.edu/mic/health-disease/skin-health/vitamin-D
Title: Vitamin D and Skin Health — **by:** Oregon State University
Website: Linus Pauling Institute Micronutrient Information Center

[s5] - https://www.nature.com/articles/s41598-024-54188-5
Author: Mehmet Ali Kallioglu, Ashutosh Sharma, Aysan Kallioglu, Sunil Kumar, Rohit Khargotra, Tej Singh — **Title:** UV index-based model for predicting synthesis of (pre-)vitamin D3 in the mediterranean basin
by: Nature Publishing Group — **Release Date:** 2024-02-12
Website: nature.com — **Publisher:** Scientific Reports

[s6] - https://www.skincancer.org/blog/sun-protection-and-vitamin-d/
Author: ANNE MARIE MCNEILL, MD, PHD and ERIN WESNER — **Title:** Sun Protection and Vitamin D
by: Skin Cancer Foundation — **Release Date:** March 14, 2019
Website: Skin Cancer Foundation

[s7] - https://www.yalemedicine.org/news/vitamin-d-myths-debunked
Author: Colleen Moriarty — **Title:** Vitamin D Myths D-bunked
by: Yale Medicine — **Release Date:** March 15, 2018
Website: Yale Medicine

[s8] - https://www.nature.com/articles/s12276-018-0038-9
Author: Sang-Min Jeon, Eun-Ae Shin — **Title:** Exploring vitamin D metabolism and function in cancer
by: Nature Publishing Group — **Release Date:** 2018-04-16
Website: nature.com — **Publisher:** Nature Publishing Group

[s9] - https://biotechnologyforbiofuels.biomedcentral.com/articles/10.1186/s13068-022-02209-8
Author: Zheyi Wang, Yan Zeng, Hongmin Jia, Niping Yang, Mengshuang Liu, Mingyue Jiang, Yanning Zheng — **Title:** Bioconversion of vitamin D3 to bioactive calcifediol and calcitriol as high-value compounds
Release Date: 13 October 2022 — **Website:** Biotechnology for Biofuels and Bioproducts
Publisher: BMC

[s10] - https://www.ncbi.nlm.nih.gov/books/NBK278935/
Author: Daniel D. Bikle, MD, PhD — **Title:** Vitamin D: Production, Metabolism and Mechanisms of Action
by: National Library of Medicine, National Institutes of Health — **Release Date:** December 31, 2021
Website: NCBI Bookshelf — **Publisher:** MDText.com, Inc.

[s11] - https://pubmed.ncbi.nlm.nih.gov/7584527/
Author: M F Holick — **Title:** Defects in the synthesis and metabolism of vitamin D
by: Boston University Medical Center — **Release Date:** 1995
Website: PubMed — **Publisher:** Exp Clin Endocrinol Diabetes

[s12] - https://clinicalepigeneticsjournal.biomedcentral.com/articles/10.1007/s13148-011-0021-y
Author: Heidrun Karlic, Franz Varga — **Title:** Impact of vitamin D metabolism on clinical epigenetics
Release Date: 08 February 2011 — **Website:** Clinical Epigenetics
Publisher: BMC

[s13] - https://www.ncbi.nlm.nih.gov/books/NBK441912/
Author: Krati Chauhan; Mahsa Shahrokhi; Martin R. Huecker — **Title:** Vitamin D
by: StatPearls Publishing — **Release Date:** 2024 Jan-
Website: NCBI Bookshelf — **Publisher:** National Library of Medicine, National Institutes of Health

[s14] - https://www.nature.com/articles/boneres201641
Author: Vaishali Veldurthy, Ran Wei, Leyla Oz, Puneet Dhawan, Yong Heui Jeon, Sylvia Christakos — **Title:** Vitamin D, calcium homeostasis and aging
by: Nature Publishing Group — **Release Date:** 2016-10-18
Website: Nature — **Publisher:** Nature Publishing Group

[s15] - https://www.ncbi.nlm.nih.gov/books/NBK482510/
Author: John J. Lofrese; Hajira Basit; Sarah L. Lappin — **Title:** Physiology, Parathyroid
by: StatPearls Publishing — **Release Date:** 2024 Jan-
Website: NCBI Bookshelf — **Publisher:** National Library of Medicine, National Institutes of Health

[s16] - https://pubmed.ncbi.nlm.nih.gov/26678915/
Author: I Szymczak, R Pawliczak — **Title:** The Active Metabolite of Vitamin D3 as a Potential Immunomodulator
Release Date: 2016-02 — **Website:** PubMed
Publisher: The Foundation for the Scandinavian Journal of Immunology

[s17] - https://pubmed.ncbi.nlm.nih.gov/26678915/
Author: I Szymczak, R Pawliczak — **Title:** The Active Metabolite of Vitamin D3 as a Potential Immunomodulator
by: Medical University of Lodz — **Release Date:** 2016-02
Website: PubMed — **Publisher:** The Foundation for the Scandinavian Journal of Immunology

[s18] - https://www.nature.com/articles/pr2009130
Author: Valencia P Walker, Robert L Modlin — **Title:** The Vitamin D Connection to Pediatric Infections and Immune Function
by: Nature Publishing Group — **Release Date:** May 2009
Website: nature.com — **Publisher:** Pediatric Research

[s19] - https://www.thieme-connect.com/products/ejournals/pdf/10.1055/s-0041-1730084.pdf
Author: Ahmed Yaqinuddin, Ayesha Rahman Ambia, Raghad A. Alaujan — **Title:** Immunomodulatory Effects of Vitamin D and Vitamin C to Improve Immunity in COVID-19 Patients
by: Alfaisal University — **Release Date:** 2021-05-12
Website: Thieme — **Publisher:** Thieme Medical and Scientific Publishers Pvt. Ltd.

[s20] - https://www.explorationpub.com/uploads/Article/A10039/10039.pdf
Author: Saptadip Samanta — **Title:** Vitamin D and immunomodulation in the skin: a useful affirmative nexus
by: Midnapore College — **Release Date:** June 30, 2021
Website: Exploration of Immunology

[s21] - https://bsd.biomedcentral.com/articles/10.1186/s13293-021-00358-3
Author: Maria Luisa Dupuis, Maria Teresa Pagano, Marina Pierdominici, Elena Ortona — **Title:** The role of vitamin D in autoimmune diseases: could sex make the difference?
by: BMC (Biomed Central) — **Release Date:** 12 January 2021
Website: Biology of Sex Differences — **Publisher:** BMC

[s22] - https://academic.oup.com/braincomms/article-pdf/4/4/fcac171/45028143/fcac171.pdf
Author: Manon Galoppin, Saniya Kari, Sasha Soldati, Arindam Pal, Manon Rival, Britta Engelhardt, Anne Astier, Eric Thouvenot — **Title:** Full spectrum of vitamin D immunomodulation in multiple sclerosis: mechanisms and therapeutic implications
by: Oxford University Press — **Release Date:** June 30, 2022
Website: Oxford Academic — **Publisher:** Oxford University Press

[s23] - https://www.nature.com/articles/s41598-024-51779-0
Author: Wei Z. Yeh, Rodney Lea, Jim Stankovich, Sandeep Sampangi, Louise Laverick, Anneke Van der Walt, Vilija Jokubaitis, Melissa Gresle, Helmut Butzkueven — **Title:** Transcriptomics identifies blunted immunomodulatory effects of vitamin D in people with multiple sclerosis
by: Nature Publishing Group — **Release Date:** 16 January 2024
Website: Nature — **Publisher:** Scientific Reports

[s24] - https://blog.bridgeathletic.com/vitamin-d-a-key-player-in-bone-health-sports-performance-recovery
Author: Dr. Emily Kraus — **Title:** Vitamin D: A Key Player in Bone Health, Sports Performance, Recovery
by: Bridge Athletic — **Release Date:** February 13, 2017
Website: Bridge Athletic

[s25] - http://www.gssiweb.org/sports-science-exchange/article/sse-148-the-importance-of-vitamin-d-for-athletes
Author: Enette Larson-Meyer — **Title:** The Importance of Vitamin D for Athletes
by: GSSI — **Release Date:** July 2015
Website: Sports Science Exchange

[s26] - https://www.ncbi.nlm.nih.gov/pmc/articles/PMC4427016/
Author: Matthieu Halfon, Olivier Phan, Daniel Teta — **Title:** Vitamin D: A Review on Its Effects on Muscle Strength, the Risk of Fall, and Frailty
by: Centre Hospitalier Universitaire Vaudois (CHUV) — **Release Date:** 2015 Apr 27
Website: NCBI — **Publisher:** Hindawi Publishing Corporation

[s27] - https://www.garvan.org.au/news-resources/news/vitamin-d-deficiency-may-impair-muscle-function
Author: Dr Andrew Philp — **Title:** Vitamin D deficiency may impair muscle function
by: Garvan Institute of Medical Research — **Release Date:** 2021-04-21
Website: Garvan Institute of Medical Research

[s28] - https://jissn.biomedcentral.com/articles/10.1186/s12970-015-0093-8
Author: Dylan T. Dahlquist, Brad P. Dieter, Michael S. Koehle — **Title:** Plausible ergogenic effects of vitamin D on athletic performance and recovery
Release Date: 19 August 2015 — **Website:** Journal of the International Society of Sports Nutrition
Publisher: BMC

[s29] - https://pubmed.ncbi.nlm.nih.gov/24256495/
Author: Christian M Girgis, Roderick J Clifton-Bligh, Nigel Turner, Sue Lynn Lau, Jenny E Gunton
Title: Effects of vitamin D in skeletal muscle: falls, strength, athletic performance and insulin sensitivity
by: Garvan Institute of Medical Research
Release Date: 2014-02
Website: PubMed
Publisher: John Wiley Sons Ltd

[s30] - https://pubmed.ncbi.nlm.nih.gov/26535872/
Author: Matthew A Wyon, Roger Wolman, Alan M Nevill, Ross Cloak, George S Metsios, Dougl as Gould, Andrew Ingham, Yiannis Koutedakis
Title: Acute Effects of Vitamin D3 Supplementation on Muscle Strength in Judoka Athletes: A Randomized Placebo-Controlled, Double-Blind Trial
Release Date: 2016-07
Website: PubMed
Publisher: Clin J Sport Med

[s31] - https://jneuroengrehab.biomedcentral.com/articles/10.1186/1743-0003-7-50
Author: Cédric Annweiler, Manuel Montero-Odasso, Anne M Schott, Gilles Berrut, Bruno Fantino, Olivier Beauchet
Title: Fall prevention and vitamin D in the elderly: an overview of the key role of the non-bone effects
Release Date: 11 October 2010
Website: Journal of NeuroEngineering and Rehabilitation
Publisher: BMC

[s32] - https://pubmed.ncbi.nlm.nih.gov/28516265/
Author: Michael F Holick
Title: The vitamin D deficiency pandemic: Appro aches for diagnosis, treatment and prevention
by: Boston University Medical Center
Release Date: 2017-06
Website: PubMed
Publisher: Springer

[s33] - https://www.nature.com/articles/s41430-020-0558-y
Author: Karin Amrein, Mario Scherkl, Magdalena H offmann, Stefan Neuwersch-Sommeregger, M arkus Kstenberger, Adelina Tmava Berisha, Gennaro Martucci, Stefan Pilz, Oliver Malle
Title: Vitamin D deficiency 2.0: an update on the current status worldwide
by: Nature Publishing Group
Release Date: 20 January 2020
Website: Nature
Publisher: European Journal of Clinical Nutrition

[s34] - https://www.yalemedicine.org/conditions/vitamin-d-deficiency
Title: Vitamin D Deficiency
by: Yale Medicine
Website: Yale Medicine

[s35] - https://lpi.oregonstate.edu/mic/vitamins/vitamin-D
Title: Vitamin D
by: Oregon State University
Website: Linus Pauling Institute

[s36] - https://bmcgeriatr.biomedcentral.com/articles/10.1186/s12877-016-0405-0
Author: Isolde Sommer, Ursula Griebler, Christina Kien, Stefanie Auer, Irma Klerings, Renate Hammer, Peter Holzer, Gerald Gartlehner
Title: Vitamin D deficiency as a risk factor for dementia: a systematic review and meta-analysis
by: BMC
Release Date: 2017-01-13
Website: BMC Geriatrics
Publisher: BMC

[s37] - https://medlineplus.gov/vitaminddeficiency.html
Title: Vitamin D Deficiency
by: National Library of Medicine
Release Date: April 22, 2024
Website: MedlinePlus

[s38] - https://www.ncbi.nlm.nih.gov/books/NBK532266/
Author: Omeed Sizar; Swapnil Khare; Amandeep Goy al; Amy Givler
Title: Vitamin D Deficiency
by: StatPearls Publishing
Release Date: 2024 Jan-
Website: NCBI Bookshelf
Publisher: StatPearls Publishing

[s39] - https://www.nature.com/articles/s41430-020-0558-y
Author: Karin Amrein, Mario Scherkl, Magdalena H offmann, Stefan Neuwersch-Sommeregger, M arkus Kstenberger, Adelina Tmava Berisha, Gennaro Martucci, Stefan Pilz, Oliver Malle
Title: Vitamin D deficiency 2.0: an update on the current status worldwide
Release Date: 20 January 2020
Website: Nature
Publisher: European Journal of Clinical Nutrition

[s40] - https://pubmed.ncbi.nlm.nih.gov/31959942/
Author: Karin Amrein, Mario Scherkl, Magdalena H offmann, Stefan Neuwersch-Sommeregger, M arkus Kstenberger, Adelina Tmava Berisha, Gennaro Martucci, Stefan Pilz, Oliver Malle
Title: Vitamin D deficiency 2.0: an update on the current status worldwide
by: Medical University of Graz
Release Date: 2020-01-20
Website: PubMed
Publisher: Eur J Clin Nutr

[s41] - https://news.tulane.edu/pr/could-vitamin-deficiency-cause-double-jointedness-and-troubling-connective-tissue-disorder
Author: Andrew J. Yawn
Title: Could a Vitamin Deficiency Cause 'double-jointedness' and Troubling Connective-tissue Disorder?
by: Tulane University
Release Date: April 10, 2023
Website: Tulane News

[s42] - https://lpi.oregonstate.edu/mic/vitamins/vitamin-D
Title: Vitamin D
by: Oregon State University
Website: Linus Pauling Institute

[s43] - https://bmcnutr.biomedcentral.com/articles/10.1186/s40795-023-00767-0
Author: Mahendra Kumar Trivedi, Alice Branton, D ahryn Trivedi, Sambhu Mondal, Snehasis Jana
Title: Vitamin D3 supplementation improves spatial memory, muscle function, pain score, and modulates different functional physiological biomarkers in vitamin D3 deficiency diet (VDD)-induced rats model
Release Date: 25 September 2023
Website: BMC Nutrition
Publisher: BMC

[s44] - https://bsd.biomedcentral.com/articles/10.1186/s13293-021-00358-3
Author: Maria Luisa Dupuis, Maria Teresa Pagano, Marina Pierdominici, Elena Ortona
Title: The role of vitamin D in autoimmune diseases: could sex make the difference?
by: BMC
Release Date: 2021-01-12
Website: Biology of Sex Differences
Publisher: BMC

[s45] - https://www.nature.com/articles/pr2009130
Author: Valencia P Walker, Robert L Modlin
Title: The Vitamin D Connection to Pediatric In fections and Immune Function
Release Date: May 2009
Website: nature.com
Publisher: Pediatric Research

[s46] - https://link.springer.com/article/10.1007/s00223-019-00577-2
Author: Stephanie R. Harrison, Danyang Li, Louisa E. Jeffery, Karim Raza, Martin Hewison | **Title:** Vitamin D, Autoimmune Disease and Rheumatoid Arthritis
by: Springer | **Release Date:** 08 July 2019
Website: SpringerLink | **Publisher:** Calcified Tissue International

[s47] - https://jneuroinflammation.biomedcentral.com/articles/10.1186/1742-2094-9-201
Author: Gehan A Mostafa, Laila Y AL-Ayadhi | **Title:** Reduced serum concentrations of 25-hydroxy vitamin D in children with autism: Relation to autoimmunity
Release Date: 17 August 2012 | **Website:** Journal of Neuroinflammation
Publisher: BMC

[s48] - https://pubmed.ncbi.nlm.nih.gov/30853311/
Author: Erin Yamamoto, Trine N Joergensen | **Title:** Immunological effects of vitamin D and their relations to autoimmunity
by: Cleveland Clinic | **Release Date:** 2019-03-08
Website: PubMed | **Publisher:** Elsevier Ltd

[s49] - https://pubmed.ncbi.nlm.nih.gov/15585788/
Author: Michael F Holick | **Title:** Sunlight and vitamin D for bone health and prevention of autoimmune diseases, cancers, and cardiovascular disease
by: Boston University Medical Center | **Release Date:** 2004-12
Website: PubMed | **Publisher:** American Journal of Clinical Nutrition

[s50] - https://www.ncbi.nlm.nih.gov/pmc/articles/PMC10379599/
Author: Mansour Almuqbil, Moneer E Almadani, Salem Ahmad Albraiki, Ali Musharraf Alamri, Ahmed Alshehri, Adel Alghamdi, Sultan Alshehri, Syed Mohammed Basheeruddin Asdaq | **Title:** Impact of Vitamin D Deficiency on Mental Health in University Students: A Cross-Sectional Study
Release Date: 2023-07-23 | **Website:** NCBI
Publisher: MDPI

[s51] - https://psychiatry-psychopharmacology.com/en/vitamin-d-deficiency-in-depressive-anxiety-and-adjustment-disorder-13722
Author: Efruz Pirdogan Aydin, Mihriban Dalkiran Varkal, Omur Gunday Toker, Omer Akil Ozer, Kayihan Oguz Karamustafalioglu | **Title:** Vitamin D deficiency in depressive, anxiety and adjustment disorder
by: Sisli Hamidiye Etfal Training and Research Hospital | **Release Date:** 13 February 2021
Website: Psychiatry and Clinical Psychopharmacology

[s52] - https://link.springer.com/article/10.1007/s13668-022-00441-0
Author: Serife Akpinar, Makbule Gezmen Karadag | **Title:** Is Vitamin D Important in Anxiety or Depression? What Is the Truth?
by: Springer | **Release Date:** 2022-09-13
Website: SpringerLink | **Publisher:** Current Nutrition Reports

[s53] - https://pubmed.ncbi.nlm.nih.gov/24226892/
Author: Lucinda J Black, Peter Jacoby, Karina L Allen, Gina S Trapp, Prue H Hart, Susan M Byrne, Trevor A Mori, Lawrence J Beilin, Wendy H Oddy | **Title:** Low vitamin D levels are associated with symptoms of depression in young adult males
by: Telethon Institute for Child Health Research, Centre for Child Health Research, The University of Western Australia | **Release Date:** 2014-05
Website: PubMed | **Publisher:** Aust N Z J Psychiatry

[s54] - https://pubmed.ncbi.nlm.nih.gov/34835934/
Author: Dominika Guzek, Aleksandra Kolota, Katarzyna Lachowicz, Dominika Skolmowska, Malgorzata Stachon, Dominika Glabska | **Title:** Influence of Vitamin D Supplementation on Mental Health in Diabetic Patients: A Systematic Review
by: Warsaw University of Life Sciences (WULS-SGGW) | **Release Date:** 2021-10-20
Website: pubmed.ncbi.nlm.nih.gov | **Publisher:** Nutrients

[s55] - https://www.nature.com/articles/s41533-021-00239-7
Author: Mohammad J. Alkhatatbeh, Haneen S. Almomani, Khalid K. Abdul-Razzak, Shaher Samrah | **Title:** Association of asthma with low serum vitamin D and its related musculoskeletal and psychological symptoms in adults: a case-control study
by: King Abdullah University Hospital | **Release Date:** 2021-05-14
Website: Nature | **Publisher:** npj Primary Care Respiratory Medicine

[s56] - https://lpi.oregonstate.edu/mic/health-disease/skin-health/vitamin-D
Title: Vitamin D and Skin Health | **by:** Oregon State University
Website: Linus Pauling Institute Micronutrient Information Center

[s57] - https://www.solius.com/benefits-of-sunlight
Title: The Health Benefits of Sunlight | **by:** Solius
Website: Solius

[s58] - https://www.nature.com/articles/s41598-017-11362-2
Author: T. A. Kalajian, A. Aldoukhi, A. J. Veronikis, K. Persons, M. F. Holick | **Title:** Ultraviolet B Light Emitting Diodes (LEDs) Are More Efficient and Effective in Producing Vitamin D3 in Human Skin Compared to Natural Sunlight
Release Date: 2017-09-13 | **Website:** Nature
Publisher: Scientific Reports

[s59] - https://www.nhs.uk/conditions/vitamins-and-minerals/vitamin-d/
Title: Vitamin D | **by:** NHS
Release Date: 03 August 2020 | **Website:** NHS

[s60] - https://ipo.rpi.edu/invention/uvb-artificial-sunlight-device-vitamin-d-production
Author: Danuel Carr, Ukwatte Lokuliyanage Indika Upendra Perera, Rohan Nagare | **Title:** UVB, Artificial Sunlight Device for Vitamin-D Production
by: Rensselaer Polytechnic Institute | **Release Date:** 14 July, 2020
Website: Rensselaer Polytechnic Institute

[s61] - https://www.skincancer.org/blog/sun-protection-and-vitamin-d/
Author: ANNE MARIE MCNEILL, MD, PHD and ERIN WESNER | **Title:** Sun Protection and Vitamin D
by: Skin Cancer Foundation | **Release Date:** March 14, 2019
Website: Skin Cancer Foundation

[s62] - https://www.nhs.uk/conditions/vitamins-and-minerals/vitamin-d/
Title: Vitamin D | **by:** NHS
Release Date: 03 August 2020 | **Website:** NHS

[s63] - https://www.nhs.uk/pregnancy/keeping-well/vitamins-supplements-and-nutrition/
Title: Vitamins, supplements and nutrition in pregnancy by: NHS
Release Date: 1 September 2023 Website: NHS

[s64] - https://www.ncbi.nlm.nih.gov/books/NBK218749/
Author: National Research Council (US) Committee on Diet and Health Title: Diet and Health: Implications for Reducing Chronic Disease Risk
Release Date: 1989 Website: NCBI
Publisher: National Academies Press (US)

[s65] - https://extension.colostate.edu/topic-areas/nutrition-food-safety-health/fat-soluble-vitamins-a-d-e-and-k-9-315/
Author: J. Clifford, A. Kozil Title: Fat-Soluble Vitamins: A, D, E, and K 9.315
by: Colorado State University Extension Release Date: 917
Website: Colorado State University Extension

[s66] - https://www.yalemedicine.org/news/vitamin-d-myths-debunked
Author: Colleen Moriarty Title: Vitamin D Myths D-bunked
by: Yale Medicine Release Date: March 15, 2018
Website: Yale Medicine

[s67] - https://www.nature.com/articles/s41430-020-0558-y
Author: Karin Amrein, Mario Scherkl, Magdalena Hoffmann, Stefan Neuwersch-Sommeregger, Markus Kstenberger, Adelina Tmava Berisha, Gennaro Martucci, Stefan Pilz, Oliver Malle Title: Vitamin D deficiency 2.0: an update on the current status worldwide
by: Nature Publishing Group Release Date: 20 January 2020
Website: Nature Publisher: European Journal of Clinical Nutrition

[s68] - https://www.nhs.uk/conditions/vitamins-and-minerals/vitamin-d/
Title: Vitamin D by: NHS
Release Date: 03 August 2020 Website: NHS

[s69] - https://www.canada.ca/en/health-canada/services/nutrients/vitamin-d.html
Title: Vitamin D by: Government of Canada
Release Date: 2022-05-02 Website: Canada.ca
Publisher: Health Canada

[s70] - https://www.ncbi.nlm.nih.gov/books/NBK218749/
Author: National Research Council (US) Committee on Diet and Health Title: Diet and Health: Implications for Reducing Chronic Disease Risk
Release Date: 1989 Website: NCBI
Publisher: National Academies Press (US)

[s71] - https://medlineplus.gov/ency/article/002399.htm
Title: Vitamins by: National Library of Medicine
Release Date: 01192023 Website: MedlinePlus
Publisher: A.D.A.M., Inc.

[s72] - https://medlineplus.gov/lab-tests/vitamin-d-test/
Title: Vitamin D Test by: National Library of Medicine
Website: MedlinePlus

[s73] - https://extension.colostate.edu/topic-areas/nutrition-food-safety-health/fat-soluble-vitamins-a-d-e-and-k-9-315/
Author: J. Clifford, A. Kozil Title: Fat-Soluble Vitamins: A, D, E, and K 9.315
by: Colorado State University Extension Release Date: 917
Website: Colorado State University Extension

[s74] - https://www.yalemedicine.org/news/vitamin-d-myths-debunked
Author: Colleen Moriarty Title: Vitamin D Myths D-bunked
by: Yale Medicine Release Date: March 15, 2018
Website: Yale Medicine

[s75] - https://www.skincancer.org/blog/sun-protection-and-vitamin-d/
Author: ANNE MARIE MCNEILL, MD, PHD and ERIN WESNER Title: Sun Protection and Vitamin D
by: The Skin Cancer Foundation Release Date: March 14, 2019
Website: Skin Cancer Foundation

[s76] - https://lpi.oregonstate.edu/mic/vitamins/vitamin-D
Title: Vitamin D by: Oregon State University
Website: Linus Pauling Institute

[s77] - https://www.foundmyfitness.com/topics/vitamin-d
Author: Rhonda Patrick Title: Vitamin D
by: FoundMyFitness Website: FoundMyFitness

[s78]
https://www.cambridge.org/core/services/aop-cambridge-core/content/view/49816B8345AFC98DB16320F12608E2A2/S0029665117000349a.pdf/vitamin-d-deficiency-as-a-public-health-issue-using-vitamin-d2-or-vitamin-d3-in-future-fortification-strategies.pdf
Author: Louise R. Wilson, Laura Tripkovic, Kathryn H. Hart, Susan A Lanham-New Title: Vitamin D deficiency as a public health issue: using vitamin D2 or vitamin D3 in future fortification strategies
by: University of Surrey Release Date: 28 March 2017
Website: Cambridge University Press Publisher: Proceedings of the Nutrition Society

[s79] - http://www.gssiweb.org/sports-science-exchange/article/sse-147-vitamin-d-measurement-supplementation-what-when-why-how-
Author: Graeme L. Close Title: Vitamin D Measurement Supplementation: What, When, Why How?
by: Gatorade Sports Science Institute (GSSI) Release Date: July 2015
Website: Sports Science Exchange

[s80] - https://www.cancer.gov/about-cancer/causes-prevention/risk/diet/vitamin-d-fact-sheet
Title: Vitamin D and Cancer by: National Cancer Institute
Release Date: May 9, 2023 Website: cancer.gov
Publisher: U.S. Department of Health and Human Services

[s81] - https://medlineplus.gov/lab-tests/vitamin-d-test/
Title: Vitamin D Test by: National Library of Medicine
Website: MedlinePlus Publisher: U.S. Department of Health and Human Services

[s82] - https://www.cancer.gov/about-cancer/causes-prevention/risk/diet/vitamin-d-fact-sheet
Title: Vitamin D and Cancer by: National Cancer Institute
Release Date: May 9, 2023 Website: cancer.gov
Publisher: U.S. Department of Health and Human Services

[s83] - https://www.yalemedicine.org/news/vitamin-d-myths-debunked
Author: Colleen Moriarty Title: Vitamin D Myths D-bunked
by: Yale Medicine Release Date: March 15, 2018
Website: Yale Medicine

[s84] - https://www.ncbi.nlm.nih.gov/books/NBK441912/

Author:	Krati Chauhan; Mahsa Shahrokhi; Martin R. Huecker	Title:	Vitamin D
by:	StatPearls Publishing	Release Date:	2024 Jan
Website:	NCBI Bookshelf	Publisher:	National Library of Medicine, National Institutes of Health

[s85] - https://pubmed.ncbi.nlm.nih.gov/10692090/

Author:	H Glerup, K Mikkelsen, L Poulsen, E Hass, S Overbeck, J Thomsen, P Charles, E F Eriksen	Title:	Commonly recommended daily intake of vitamin D is not sufficient if sunlight exposure is limited
by:	University Hospital of Aarhus	Release Date:	2000-02
Website:	PubMed	Publisher:	J Intern Med

[s86] - https://www.nature.com/articles/s41430-020-0558-y

Author:	Karin Amrein, Mario Scherkl, Magdalena Hoffmann, Stefan Neuwersch-Sommeregger, Markus Kstenberger, Adelina Tmava Berisha, Gennaro Martucci, Stefan Pilz, Oliver Malle	Title:	Vitamin D deficiency 2.0: an update on the current status worldwide
by:	Nature Publishing Group	Release Date:	20 January 2020
Website:	Nature	Publisher:	European Journal of Clinical Nutrition

[s87] - https://www.canada.ca/en/health-canada/services/drugs-health-products/drug-products/prescription-drug-list/notices-changes/notice-amendment-vitamin-d.html

Title:	Notice: Prescription Drug List (PDL): Vitamin D	by:	Health Canada
Release Date:	2021-02-22	Website:	Canada.ca

[s88] - https://pubmed.ncbi.nlm.nih.gov/15225842/

Author:	Reinhold Vieth	Title:	Why the optimal requirement for Vitamin D3 is probably much higher than what is officially recommended for adults
Release Date:	2004-05	Website:	PubMed
Publisher:	J Steroid Biochem Mol Biol		

[s89] - https://www.nhs.uk/conditions/vitamins-and-minerals/vitamin-d/

Title:	Vitamin D	by:	NHS
Release Date:	03 August 2020	Website:	NHS

[s90] - https://pubmed.ncbi.nlm.nih.gov/18977996/

Author:	Carol L Wagner, Frank R Greer	Title:	Prevention of rickets and vitamin D deficiency in infants, children, and adolescents
by:	American Academy of Pediatrics	Release Date:	2008-11
Website:	PubMed	Publisher:	Pediatrics

[s91] - https://www.rnoh.nhs.uk/services/children-and-adolescents/vitamin-d-children

Title:	Vitamin D in Children	by:	RNOH NHS
Website:	RNOH NHS		

[s92] - https://www.canada.ca/en/health-canada/services/drugs-health-products/drug-products/prescription-drug-list/notices-changes/notice-amendment-vitamin-d.html

Title:	Notice: Prescription Drug List (PDL): Vitamin D	by:	Health Canada
Release Date:	2021-02-22	Website:	Canada.ca
Publisher:	Government of Canada		

[s93] - https://pubmed.ncbi.nlm.nih.gov/20229973/

Author:	Catherine F Casey, David C Slawson, Lindsey R Neal	Title:	Vitamin D supplementation in infants, children, and adolescents
Release Date:	2010-03-15	Website:	PubMed
Publisher:	American Family Physician		

[s94] - https://lpi.oregonstate.edu/mic/life-stages/older-adults

Title:	Micronutrients for Older Adults	by:	Oregon State University
Website:	Linus Pauling Institute		

[s95] - https://bmcgeriatr.biomedcentral.com/articles/10.1186/s12877-024-05009-x

Author:	Long Tan, Ruiqian He, Xiaoxue Zheng	Title:	Effect of vitamin D, calcium, or combined supplementation on fall prevention: a systematic review and updated network meta-analysis
by:	BMC	Release Date:	2024-05-02
Website:	BMC Geriatrics	Publisher:	BMC

[s96] - https://article.imrpress.com/journal/IJVNR/81/4/10.1024/0300-9831/a000072/7638179ac4c524021b0229b0659b5c7d.pdf

Author:	Heike Bischoff-Ferrari, Hannes B. Sthelin, Paul Walter	Title:	Vitamin D Effects on Bone and Muscle
by:	Hogrefe AG	Release Date:	2011
Website:	International Journal of Vitamin and Nutrition Research	Publisher:	Hans Huber Publishers

[s97] - https://link.springer.com/article/10.1007/s00198-016-3833-y

Author:	H. Hin, J. Tomson, C. Newman, R. Kurien, M. Lay, J. Cox, J. Sayer, M. Hill, J. Emberson, J. Armitage, R. Clarke	Title:	Optimum dose of vitamin D for disease prevention in older people: BEST-D trial of vitamin D in primary care
by:	Springer	Release Date:	2016-12-16
Website:	SpringerLink	Publisher:	Osteoporosis International

[s98] - https://pubmed.ncbi.nlm.nih.gov/17151835/

Author:	H A Bischoff-Ferrari	Title:	How to select the doses of vitamin D in the management of osteoporosis
Release Date:	2007-04	Website:	PubMed
Publisher:	Osteoporosis International		

[s99] - https://thischangedmypractice.com/correct-dosing-for-vit-d/

Author:	Dr. Kenneth Madden	Title:	What is the correct dosing for Vitamin D?
by:	The University of British Columbia	Release Date:	December 6, 2011
Website:	This Changed My Practice	Publisher:	UBC CPD

[s100] - https://betterhealthwhileaging.net/vitamin-d-healthy-aging-dose-faqs/

Author:	Leslie Kernisan, MD MPH	Title:	Vitamin D: What to Know (Why to Be Careful About High Doses)
by:	Better Health While Aging	Release Date:	June 2024
Website:	Better Health While Aging		

[s101] - https://www.nature.com/articles/s41430-020-0558-y
Author: Karin Amrein, Mario Scherkl, Magdalena Hoffmann, Stefan Neuwersch-Sommeregger, Markus Kstenberger, Adelina Tmava Berisha, Gennaro Martucci, Stefan Pilz, Oliver Malle Title: Vitamin D deficiency 2.0: an update on the current status worldwide
Release Date: 20 January 2020   Website: Nature
Publisher: European Journal of Clinical Nutrition

[s102] - https://www.gov.scot/publications/vitamin-d-advice-for-parents/
Title: Vitamin D: advice for parents   by: Scottish Government
Release Date: 27 July 2023   Website: Scottish Government

[s103] - https://pubmed.ncbi.nlm.nih.gov/32487800/
Author: Faustino R Perez-Lopez, Stefan Pilz, Peter Chedraui   Title: Vitamin D supplementation during pregnancy: an overview
Release Date: 2020-10   Website: PubMed
Publisher: Curr Opin Obstet Gynecol

[s104] - https://www.nature.com/articles/boneres201730
Author: Bruce W Hollis, Carol L Wagner   Title: New insights into the vitamin D requirements during pregnancy
by: Nature Publishing Group   Release Date: 29 August 2017
Website: nature.com   Publisher: Nature Publishing Group

[s105] - https://www.nhs.uk/pregnancy/keeping-well/vitamins-supplements-and-nutrition/
Title: Vitamins, supplements and nutrition in pregnancy   by: NHS
Release Date: 2023-09-01   Website: NHS

[s106] - https://www.nhs.uk/conditions/vitamins-and-minerals/vitamin-d/
Title: Vitamin D   by: NHS
Release Date: 03 August 2020   Website: NHS

[s107] https://www.bluecrossnc.com/content/dam/bcbsnc/pdf/providers/policies-guidelines-codes/policies/commercial/laboratory/vitamin_d_testing.pdf
Title: Vitamin D Testing AHS G2005   by: Blue Cross Blue Shield of North Carolina
Release Date: 01012019   Website: Blue Cross Blue Shield of North Carolina

[s108] - https://link.springer.com/article/10.1007/s11154-021-09693-7
Author: John P. Bilezikian, Anna Maria Formenti, Robert A. Adler, Neil Binkley, Roger Bouillon, Marise Lazaretti-Castro, Claudio Marcocci, Nicola Napoli, Rene Rizzoli, Andrea Giustina   Title: Vitamin D: Dosing, levels, form, and route of administration: Does one approach fit all?
by: Springer   Release Date: 2021-12-23
Website: SpringerLink   Publisher: Springer

[s109] - https://med.virginia.edu/ginutrition/wp-content/uploads/sites/199/2021/06/May-2021-Vitamin-D-Replacement.pdf
Author: Ronak M. Patel, M.D., Lindsay Bazydlo, Ph.D., Sue A. Brown, M.D., Alan C. Dalkin, M.D.   Title: Vitamin D Replacement in Adults: Current Strategies in Clinical Management
by: University of Virginia Health System   Release Date: May 2021
Website: University of Virginia Health System   Publisher: Practical Gastroenterology

[s110] - https://www.ncbi.nlm.nih.gov/books/NBK441912/
Author: Krati Chauhan; Mahsa Shahrokhi; Martin R. Huecker   Title: Vitamin D
by: StatPearls Publishing   Release Date: 2024 Jan-
Website: NCBI Bookshelf   Publisher: National Library of Medicine, National Institutes of Health

[s111] - https://link.springer.com/article/10.1007/s11154-021-09693-7
Author: John P. Bilezikian, Anna Maria Formenti, Robert A. Adler, Neil Binkley, Roger Bouillon, Marise Lazaretti-Castro, Claudio Marcocci, Nicola Napoli, Rene Rizzoli, Andrea Giustina   Title: Vitamin D: Dosing, levels, form, and route of administration: Does one approach fit all?
Release Date: 23 December 2021   Website: SpringerLink
Publisher: Springer

[s112] https://www.med.unc.edu/pediatrics/cccp/wp-content/uploads/sites/1156/gravity_forms/1-c06e424ddddee8826f29e1bc5926a251/2021/06/Stoss-Therapy-Guidelines-FINAL.pdf
Title: High-Dose Vitamin D3 (Stoss Therapy) Use in Cystic Fibrosis Patients   by: UNC Medical Center
Release Date: January 2021   Website: University of North Carolina at Chapel Hill

[s113] - https://www2.gov.bc.ca/gov/content/health/practitioner-professional-resources/bc-guidelines/vitamin-d-testing
Title: Vitamin D Testing   by: Government of British Columbia
Release Date: June 3, 2024   Website: Government of British Columbia

[s114] https://www.bluecrossnc.com/content/dam/bcbsnc/pdf/providers/policies-guidelines-codes/policies/commercial/laboratory/vitamin_d_testing.pdf
Title: Vitamin D Testing AHS G2005   by: Blue Cross Blue Shield of North Carolina
Release Date: 01012019   Website: Blue Cross Blue Shield of North Carolina

[s115] - https://www.nhs.uk/conditions/vitamins-and-minerals/vitamin-d/
Title: Vitamin D   by: NHS
Release Date: 03 August 2020   Website: NHS

[s116] - https://www.ncbi.nlm.nih.gov/books/NBK548094/
Title: Vitamin D   by: National Institute of Diabetes and Digestive and Kidney Diseases
Release Date: 2021-05-27   Website: NCBI Bookshelf
Publisher: National Library of Medicine

[s117] - https://pubmed.ncbi.nlm.nih.gov/36853379/
Author: Armin Zittermann, Christian Trummer, Verena Theiler-Schwetz, Stefan Pilz   Title: Long-term supplementation with 3200 to 4000 IU of vitamin D daily and adverse events: a systematic review and meta-analysis of randomized controlled trials
Release Date: 2023-02-28   Website: PubMed
Publisher: Eur J Nutr

[s118] - https://www.cancer.gov/about-cancer/causes-prevention/risk/diet/vitamin-d-fact-sheet
Title: Vitamin D and Cancer   by: National Cancer Institute
Release Date: May 9, 2023   Website: cancer.gov
Publisher: U.S. Department of Health and Human Services

[s119] - https://www.nature.com/articles/s41430-020-0558-y
Author: Karin Amrein, Mario Scherkl, Magdalena Hoffmann, Stefan Neuwersch-Sommeregger, Markus Kstenberger, Adelina Tmava Berisha, Gennaro Martucci, Stefan Pilz, Oliver Malle
Title: Vitamin D deficiency 2.0: an update on the current status worldwide
by: Nature Publishing Group
Release Date: 20 January 2020
Website: nature.com
Publisher: European Journal of Clinical Nutrition

[s120] - https://www.nps.org.au/assets/AP/pdf/p119-Moses.pdf
Author: Geraldine Moses AM
Title: The safety of commonly used vitamins and minerals
by: NPS MedicineWise
Release Date: August 2021
Website: NPS MedicineWise
Publisher: Australian Prescriber

[s121] - https://www.betterhealth.vic.gov.au/health/healthyliving/vitamin-and-mineral-supplements-what-to-know
Author: Melissa Burton
Title: Vitamin and mineral supplements - what to know
by: Deakin University
Release Date: 2024-05-14
Website: Better Health Channel
Publisher: Department of Health and Human Services, Victoria

[s122]
https://www.med.unc.edu/pediatrics/cccp/wp-content/uploads/sites/1156/gravity_forms/1-c06e424ddddee8826f29e1bc5926a251/2021/06/Stoss-Therapy-Guidelines-FINAL.pdf
Title: High-Dose Vitamin D3 (Stoss Therapy) Use in Cystic Fibrosis Patients
by: UNC Medical Center
Release Date: January 2021
Website: University of North Carolina at Chapel Hill

[s123] - https://www.ncbi.nlm.nih.gov/books/NBK441912/
Author: Krati Chauhan; Mahsa Shahrokhi; Martin R. Huecker
Title: Vitamin D
by: StatPearls Publishing
Release Date: 2024 Jan-
Website: NCBI Bookshelf
Publisher: National Library of Medicine, National Institutes of Health

[s124] - https://kdigo.org/wp-content/uploads/2017/02/2017-KDIGO-CKD-MBD-GL-Update.pdf
Title: KDIGO 2017 Clinical Practice Guideline Update for the Diagnosis, Evaluation, Prevention, and Treatment of Chronic Kidney DiseaseMineral and Bone Disorder (CKD-MBD)
by: KDIGO
Release Date: July 2017
Website: www.kisupplements.org
Publisher: Kidney International Supplements

[s125] - https://www2.gov.bc.ca/gov/content/health/practitioner-professional-resources/bc-guidelines/vitamin-d-testing
Title: Vitamin D Testing
by: Government of British Columbia
Release Date: June 3, 2024
Website: Government of British Columbia

[s126] - https://tp.amegroups.org/article/view/22713/html
Author: Natalie G. Martin, Tarah Rigterink, Mustafa Adamji, Catherine L. Wall, Andrew S. Day
Title: Single high-dose oral vitamin D3 treatment in New Zealand children with inflammatory bowel disease
by: University of Otago Christchurch
Release Date: January 28, 2019
Website: tp.amegroups.org
Publisher: AME Publishing Company

[s127] - https://labeling.pfizer.com/showlabeling.aspx?id=522
Title: DEPO-PROVERA (medroxyprogesterone acetate) injection, suspension
by: Pharmacia Upjohn Company LLC
Website: Pfizer

[s128] - https://www.health.com/vitamin-d-and-k-8427006
Author: Ruth Jessen Hickman, MD
Title: Can You Take Vitamin D and Vitamin K Together?
by: Health
Release Date: January 27, 2024
Website: Health
Publisher: Dotdash Meredith

[s129]
https://www.canada.ca/en/health-canada/services/drugs-health-products/drug-products/prescription-drug-list/notices-changes/notice-amendment-vitamin-d.html
Title: Notice: Prescription Drug List (PDL): Vitamin D
by: Health Canada
Release Date: 2021-02-22
Website: Canada.ca
Publisher: Government of Canada

[s130] - https://medlineplus.gov/lab-tests/vitamin-d-test/
Title: Vitamin D Test
by: National Library of Medicine
Website: MedlinePlus

[s131] - https://link.springer.com/article/10.1007/s40261-021-01113-7
Author: Milko Radicioni, Carol Caverzasio, Stefano Rovati, Andrea Maria Giori, Irma Cupone, Fabio Marra, Giuseppe Mautone
Title: Comparative Bioavailability Study of a New Vitamin D3 Orodispersible Film Versus a Marketed Oral Solution in Healthy Volunteers
by: IBSA, Italy; Abiogen Pharma S.p.A., Italy
Release Date: 16 January 2022
Website: SpringerLink
Publisher: Springer

[s132] - https://www.yalemedicine.org/news/vitamin-d-myths-debunked
Author: Colleen Moriarty
Title: Vitamin D Myths D-bunked
by: Yale Medicine
Release Date: March 15, 2018
Website: Yale Medicine

[s133] - https://www.nhs.uk/conditions/vitamins-and-minerals/vitamin-d/
Title: Vitamin D
by: NHS
Release Date: 03 August 2020
Website: NHS

[s134] - http://www.gssiweb.org/sports-science-exchange/article/sse-148-the-importance-of-vitamin-d-for-athletes
Author: Enette Larson-Meyer
Title: The Importance of Vitamin D for Athletes
by: GSSI
Release Date: July 2015
Website: Sports Science Exchange

[s135] - https://pubmed.ncbi.nlm.nih.gov/34202578/
Author: Shaun Sabico, Mushira A Enani, Eman Sheshah, Naji J Aljohani, Dara A Aldisi, Naif H Alotaibi, Naemah Alshingetti, Suliman Y Alomar, Abdullah M Alnaami, Osama E Amer, Syed D Hussain, Nasser M Al-Daghri
Title: Effects of a 2-Week 5000 IU versus 1000 IU Vitamin D3 Supplementation on Recovery of Symptoms in Patients with Mild to Moderate Covid-19: A Randomized Clinical Trial
by: King Saud University
Release Date: 2021-06-24
Website: pubmed.ncbi.nlm.nih.gov
Publisher: Nutrients

[s136] - https://pubmed.ncbi.nlm.nih.gov/23427007/
Author: Bess Dawson-Hughes, Susan S Harris, Nancy J Palermo, Lisa Ceglia, Helen Rasmussen
Title: Meal conditions affect the absorption of supplemental vitamin D3 but not the plasma 25-hydroxyvitamin D response to supplementation
by: Jean Mayer United States Department of Agriculture Human Nutrition Research Center on Aging at Tufts University
Release Date: 2013-08
Website: PubMed
Publisher: American Society for Bone and Mineral Research

[s137] - https://www.health.com/mind-body/calcium-and-vitamin-d-supplements
Author: Maggie ONeill
Title: Can You Take Vitamin D and Calcium Together?
by: Health
Release Date: September 6, 2023
Website: Health
Publisher: Dotdash Meredith

[s138] https://www.quora.com/When-is-the-best-time-to-take-a-vitamin-D-pill-supplement-Can-I-take-it-at-night-before-bed-Should-I-take-it-with-food-If-so-what-kind-of-food-and-how-much-The-specific-vitamin-D-pill-supplement-I-am-taking-is-Vitamin-Code-RAW-D3-of-5-000-IU
Title: When is the best time to take a vitamin D pillsupplement? Can I take it at night before bed? Should I take it with food? If so, what kind of food, and how much? The specific vitamin D pillsupplement I am taking is Vitamin Code RAW D3 of 5,000 IU.
by: Quora
Website: Quora

[s139] https://medicine.umich.edu/sites/default/files/content/downloads/Williams%2C%20Christa%20December%207%202018%20Vitamin%20D.pdf
Author: Christa Williams MD
Title: The Case for Vitamin D Supplementation: Summary of the Evidence and Recommendations
by: University of Michigan
Release Date: December 7, 2018
Website: University of Michigan

[s140] - https://thenaturaldoctor.org/wp-content/uploads/2023/01/Vitamins-D3-and-K2-Another-Dynamic-Duo-By-Dr-Eccles.pdf
Author: Dr Nyjon K. Eccles BSc MBBS MRCP PhD
Title: Vitamins D3 and K2 Another Dynamic Duo!
by: The Natural Doctor
Website: thenaturaldoctor.org

[s141] - https://www.health.com/vitamin-d-and-k-8427006
Author: Ruth Jessen Hickman, MD
Title: Can You Take Vitamin D and Vitamin K Together?
by: Health
Release Date: January 27, 2024
Website: Health
Publisher: Dotdash Meredith

[s142] - https://pubmed.ncbi.nlm.nih.gov/32060566/
Author: Yingfeng Zhang, Zhipeng Liu, Lili Duan, Yeyu Ji, Sen Yang, Yuan Zhang, Hongyin Li, Yu Wang, Peng Wang, Jiepeng Chen, Ying Li
Title: Effect of Low-Dose Vitamin K2 Supplementation on Bone Mineral Density in Middle-Aged and Elderly Chinese: A Randomized Controlled Study
by: Harbin Medical University, Shenyang Pharmaceutical University
Release Date: 2020-02-14
Website: pubmed.ncbi.nlm.nih.gov
Publisher: Calcified Tissue International

[s143] - https://dmsjournal.biomedcentral.com/articles/10.1186/s13098-020-00580-w
Author: J. I. Aguayo-Ruiz, T. A. Garcia-Cobin, S. Pascoe-Gonzalez, S. Sanchez-Enriquez, I. M. Llamas-Covarrubias, T. Garcia-Iglesias, A. Lopez-Quintero, M. A. Llamas-Covarrubias, J. Trujillo-Quiroz, E. A. Rivera-Leon
Title: Effect of supplementation with vitamins D3 and K2 on undercarboxylated osteocalcin and insulin serum levels in patients with type 2 diabetes mellitus: a randomized, double-blind, clinical trial
Release Date: 2020-08-18
Publisher: BMC
Website: Diabetology Metabolic Syndrome

[s144] - https://josr-online.biomedcentral.com/articles/10.1186/s13018-021-02728-4
Author: Liyou Hu, Jindou Ji, Dong Li, Jing Meng, Bo Yu
Title: The combined effect of vitamin K and calcium on bone mineral density in humans: a meta-analysis of randomized controlled trials
Release Date: 2021-10-14
Publisher: BMC
Website: Journal of Orthopaedic Surgery and Research

[s145] - https://pdfs.semanticscholar.org/34b1/bac2241b8001f15bbb0e92c9c6cd233061fb.pdf
Author: Zane Temova Rakusa, Mitja Pislar, Albin Kristl, Robert Roskar
Title: Comprehensive Stability Study of Vitamin D3 in Aqueous Solutions and Liquid Commercial Products
by: MDPI
Release Date: 2021-04-25
Website: Pharmaceutics
Publisher: MDPI, Basel, Switzerland

[s146] - https://pubmed.ncbi.nlm.nih.gov/31156916/
Author: Zane Temova, Robert Roskar
Title: Shelf life after opening of prescription medicines and supplements with vitamin D3 for paediatric use
Release Date: 2017-03
Publisher: Eur J Hosp Pharm
Website: PubMed

[s147] - https://consensus.app/questions/are-vitamins-still-good-after-expiration-date/
Title: Are vitamins still good after expiration date
by: Consensus
Website: Consensus

[s148] - https://www.biochemia-medica.com/en/journal/23/3/10.11613/BM.2013.039
Author: Ayfer Colak, Burak Toprak, Nese Dogan, Fusun Ustuner
Title: Effect of sample type, centrifugation and storage conditions on vitamin D concentration
by: Tepecik Training and Research Hospital
Release Date: 2013-10-15
Website: Biochemia Medica

[s149] - https://nutritionandmetabolism.biomedcentral.com/articles/10.1186/1743-7075-3-36
Author: Helen A Valsamis, Surender K Arora, Barbara Labban, Samy I McFarlane
Title: Antiepileptic drugs and bone metabolism
Release Date: 06 September 2006
Publisher: BMC
Website: Nutrition Metabolism

[s150] - https://cmbl.biomedcentral.com/articles/10.1186/s11658-022-00371-3
Author: Bo Liang, George Burley, Shu Lin, Yan-Chuan Shi
Title: Osteoporosis pathogenesis and treatment: existing and emerging avenues
by: BMC
Release Date: 2022-09-04
Website: Cellular Molecular Biology Letters
Publisher: BMC

[s151] - https://medlineplus.gov/ency/article/002062.htm
Title: Calcium and bones
by: A.D.A.M., Inc.
Release Date: 06012025
Website: MedlinePlus
Publisher: National Library of Medicine

[s152] - https://www.ecmjournal.org/papers/vol035/pdf/v035a25.pdf
Author: V. Fischer, M. Haffner-Luntzer, M. Amling, A. Ignatius
Title: Calcium and vitamin D in fracture healing and post-traumatic bone turnover
Release Date: 2018
Website: European Cells and Materials

[s153] - https://pubmed.ncbi.nlm.nih.gov/15585788/
Author: Michael F Holick
Title: Sunlight and vitamin D for bone health and prevention of autoimmune diseases, cancers, and cardiovascular disease
by: Boston University Medical Center
Release Date: 2004-12
Website: PubMed
Publisher: American Journal of Clinical Nutrition

[s154] - https://pubmed.ncbi.nlm.nih.gov/11684396/
Author: P Weber
Title: Vitamin K and bone health
by: F. Hoffmann-La Roche Ltd
Release Date: 2001-10
Website: PubMed
Publisher: Nutrition

[s155] - https://josr-online.biomedcentral.com/articles/10.1186/s13018-023-04320-4
Author: Yanqi Li, Pengfei Zhao, Biyun Jiang, Kangyong Liu, Lei Zhang, Haotian Wang, Yansheng Tian, Kun Li, Guoqi Liu
Title: Modulation of the vitamin D vitamin D receptor system in osteoporosis pathogenesis: insights and therapeutic approaches
Release Date: 2023-11-13
Website: Journal of Orthopaedic Surgery and Research
Publisher: BMC

[s156] - https://www.nature.com/articles/boneres201641
Author: Vaishali Veldurthy, Ran Wei, Leyla Oz, Puneet Dhawan, Yong Heui Jeon, Sylvia Christakos
Title: Vitamin D, calcium homeostasis and aging
by: Nature Publishing Group
Release Date: 2016-10-18
Website: Nature
Publisher: Nature Publishing Group

[s157] - https://www.ncbi.nlm.nih.gov/pmc/articles/PMC10175743/
Author: Haiwei Wang, Yuchuan Luo, Haisheng Wang, Feifei Li, Fanyuan Yu, Ling Ye
Title: Mechanistic advances in osteoporosis et anti-osteoporosis therapiae
by: Sichuan University
Release Date: 2023 May 11
Website: NCBI
Publisher: Sichuan International Medical Exchange Promotion Association (SCIMEA) and John Wiley Sons Australia, Ltd.

[s158] - https://pubmed.ncbi.nlm.nih.gov/26510847/
Author: C M Weaver, D D Alexander, C J Boushey, B Dawson-Hughes, J M Lappe, M S LeBoff, S Liu, A C Looker, T C Wallace, D D Wang
Title: Calcium plus vitamin D supplementation and risk of fractures: an updated meta-analysis from the National Osteoporosis Foundation
by: National Osteoporosis Foundation
Release Date: 2015-10-28
Website: PubMed
Publisher: Osteoporosis International

[s159] - https://bmcgeriatr.biomedcentral.com/articles/10.1186/s12877-024-05009-x
Author: Long Tan, Ruiqian He, Xiaoxue Zheng
Title: Effect of vitamin D, calcium, or combined supplementation on fall prevention: a systematic review and updated network meta-analysis
by: BMC Geriatrics
Release Date: 2024-05-02
Website: BMC Geriatrics
Publisher: BioMed Central

[s160] - https://strwebprdmedia.blob.core.windows.net/media/ef2ideu2/ros-vitamin-d-and-bone-health-in-adults-february-2020.pdf
Author: Prof. Roger Francis, Dr. Terry Aspray, Prof. William Fraser, Prof. Helen Macdonald, Dr. Sanjeev Patel, Dr. Alexandra Mavroeidi, Dr. Inez Schoenmakers, Prof. Mike Stone
Title: Vitamin D and Bone Health: A Practical Clinical Guideline for Patient Management
by: Royal Osteoporosis Society
Release Date: December 2018
Website: theros.org.uk

[s161] - https://www.nogg.org.uk/full-guideline/section-5-non-pharmacological-management-osteoporosis
Title: Section 5: Non-pharmacological management of osteoporosis
by: NOGG
Website: NOGG

[s162] - https://www.ncbi.nlm.nih.gov/pmc/articles/PMC8979902/
Author: Celia L Gregson, David J Armstrong, Jean Bowden, Cyrus Cooper, John Edwards, Neil J L Gittoes, Nicholas Harvey, John Kanis, Sarah Leyland, Rebecca Low, Eugene McCloskey, Katie Moss, Jane Parker, Zoe Paskins, Kenneth Poole, David M Reid, Mike Stone, Julia Thomson, Nic Vine, Juliet Compston
Title: UK clinical guideline for the prevention and treatment of osteoporosis
by: National Osteoporosis Guideline Group (NOGG)
Release Date: 2022-04-05
Website: NCBI
Publisher: Arch Osteoporos

[s163] - https://www2.gov.bc.ca/gov/content/health/practitioner-professional-resources/bc-guidelines/osteoporosis
Title: Osteoporosis: Diagnosis, Treatment and Fracture Prevention
by: Government of British Columbia
Release Date: September 17, 2023
Website: Government of British Columbia

[s164] - https://link.springer.com/article/10.1007/s00198-015-3386-5
Author: C. M. Weaver, D. D. Alexander, C. J. Boushey, B. Dawson-Hughes, J. M. Lappe, M. S. LeBoff, S. Liu, A. C. Looker, T. C. Wallace, D. D. Wang
Title: Calcium plus vitamin D supplementation and risk of fractures: an updated meta-analysis from the National Osteoporosis Foundation
by: National Osteoporosis Foundation
Release Date: 28 October 2015
Website: SpringerLink
Publisher: Osteoporosis International

[s165] - https://e-cnr.org/DOIx.php?id=10.7762/cnr.2015.4.1.1
Author: Judith A. Beto
Title: The Role of Calcium in Human Aging
by: Loyola University Healthcare System, Dominican University
Release Date: January 16, 2015
Website: Clinical Nutrition Research
Publisher: The Korean Society of Clinical Nutrition

[s166] - https://lpi.oregonstate.edu/mic/vitamins/vitamin-D
Title: Vitamin D
by: Oregon State University
Website: Linus Pauling Institute

[s167] - https://www.esceo.org/sites/esceo/files/pdf/Rizzoli-Biver2020_Article_AreProbioticsTheNewCalciumAndV.pdf
Author: Ren Rizzoli, Emmanuel Biver
Title: Are Probiotics the New Calcium and Vitamin D for Bone Health?
by: Springer Science+Business Media, LLC
Release Date: 2020
Website: ESCEO
Publisher: Springer Nature

[s168] - https://pubmed.ncbi.nlm.nih.gov/32285249/
Author: Ren Rizzoli, Emmanuel Biver | **Title:** Are Probiotics the New Calcium and Vitamin D for Bone Health?
by: Geneva University Hospitals and Faculty of Medicine | **Release Date:** 2020-06
Website: PubMed | **Publisher:** Current Osteoporosis Reports

[s169] - https://nutritionandmetabolism.biomedcentral.com/articles/10.1186/s12986-023-00726-3
Author: Tianshu Liu, Hai Yu, Shuai Wang, Huimin Li, Xinyiran Du, Xiaodong He | **Title:** Chondroitin sulfate alleviates osteoporosis caused by calcium deficiency by regulating lipid metabolism
by: BMC Nutrition Metabolism | **Release Date:** 06 February 2023
Website: Nutrition Metabolism | **Publisher:** BMC

[s170] - https://publichealthreviews.biomedcentral.com/articles/10.1186/s40985-017-0066-3
Author: M Fiscaletti, P Stewart, CF Munns | **Title:** The importance of vitamin D in maternal and child health: a global perspective
by: BMC | **Release Date:** 01 September 2017
Website: Public Health Reviews | **Publisher:** BMC

[s171] - https://epi.alaska.gov/bulletins/docs/rr2018_04.pdf
Author: Madison Pachoe, Joe McLaughlin, MD, MPH, Rosalyn Singleton, MD, MPH, Rachel Lescher, MD, Tim Thomas, MD, Jay Butler, MD, David Compton, MD, Joe Klejka, MD, Coleman Cutchins, PharmD, Matt Hirschfeld, MD, PhD, Rebecca Morisse, RN, MPH, Jared Parrish, PhD, MPH, Deanna Stang, RN, Kenneth Thummel, PhD, Leanne Ward, MD | **Title:** Vitamin D Supplementation and Screening for the Prevention of Rickets and Osteomalacia in Alaska
by: Alaska Division of Public Health | **Release Date:** September 12, 2018
Website: Alaska Department of Health and Social Services

[s172] - https://www.e-cep.org/m/journal/view.php?number=20125555493
Author: Ju Sun Heo, MD, PhD; Young Min Ahn, MD, PhD; Ai-Rhan Ellen Kim, MD, PhD; Son Moon Shin, MD, PhD | **Title:** Breastfeeding and vitamin D
by: Korean Society of Breastfeeding Medicine | **Release Date:** December 14, 2021
Website: Korean Journal of Pediatrics | **Publisher:** Korean Pediatric Society

[s173] - https://www.indianpediatrics.net/july2017/567.pdf
Author: Anuradha Khadilkar, Vaman Khadilkar, Jagdish Chinnappa, Narendra Rathi, Rajesh Khadgawat, S Balasubramanian, Bakul Parekh, Pramod Jog | **Title:** Prevention and Treatment of Vitamin D and Calcium Deficiency in Children and Adolescents: Indian Academy of Pediatrics (IAP) Guidelines
by: Indian Academy of Pediatrics | **Release Date:** July 15, 2017
Website: Indian Pediatrics

[s174] - https://www.ncbi.nlm.nih.gov/books/NBK532266/
Author: Omeed Sizar; Swapnil Khare; Amandeep Goyal; Amy Givler | **Title:** Vitamin D Deficiency
by: StatPearls Publishing | **Release Date:** 2024 Jan
Website: NCBI Bookshelf | **Publisher:** StatPearls Publishing

[s175] - https://www.solius.com/vitamin-d-immune-system
Title: The Role of Vitamin D in the Immune System | **by:** Solius
Website: Solius

[s176] - https://www.ncbi.nlm.nih.gov/pmc/articles/PMC9954268/
Author: Hasti Gholami, John A Chmiel, Jeremy P Burton, Saman Maleki Vareki | **Title:** The Role of Microbiota-Derived Vitamins in Immune Homeostasis and Enhancing Cancer Immunotherapy
by: Western University, Lawson Health Research Institute | **Release Date:** 2023-02-18
Website: NCBI | **Publisher:** MDPI

[s177] - https://gutpathogens.biomedcentral.com/articles/10.1186/s13099-020-00385-2
Author: Samir Jawhara | **Title:** How to boost the immune defence prior to respiratory virus infections with the special focus on coronavirus infections
Release Date: 12 October 2020 | **Website:** Gut Pathogens
Publisher: BMC

[s178] - https://pubmed.ncbi.nlm.nih.gov/16373990/
Author: Eva S Wintergerst, Silvia Maggini, Dietrich H Hornig | **Title:** Immune-enhancing role of vitamin C and zinc and effect on clinical conditions
by: Bayer Consumer Care Ltd. | **Release Date:** 2005-12-21
Website: PubMed | **Publisher:** S. Karger AG, Basel

[s179] - https://link.springer.com/article/10.1007/s11154-021-09679-5
Author: Aiten Ismailova, John H. White | **Title:** Vitamin D, infections and immunity
by: Springer | **Release Date:** 29 July 2021
Website: SpringerLink | **Publisher:** Springer

[s180] - https://www.ncbi.nlm.nih.gov/pmc/articles/PMC8155592/
Author: Hassan A Alhazmi, Asim Najmi, Sadique A Javed, Shahnaz Sultana, Mohammed Al Bratty, Hafiz A Makeen, Abdulkarim M Meraya, Waquar Ahsan, Syam Mohan, Manal M E Taha, Asaad Khalid | **Title:** Medicinal Plants and Isolated Molecules Demonstrating Immunomodulation Activity as Potential Alternative Therapies for Viral Diseases Including COVID-19
by: Jazan University | **Release Date:** 2021-05-13
Website: NCBI | **Publisher:** Frontiers in Immunology

[s181] - https://www.nature.com/articles/pr2009130
Author: Valencia P Walker, Robert L Modlin | **Title:** The Vitamin D Connection to Pediatric Infections and Immune Function
Release Date: May 2009 | **Website:** nature.com
Publisher: Pediatric Research

[s182] - https://www.nature.com/articles/s41541-024-00909-w
Author: Himanshu Singh Saroha, Swati Bhat, Liza Das, Pinaki Dutta, Michael F. Holick, Naresh Sachdeva, Raman Kumar Marwaha | **Title:** Calcifediol boosts efficacy of ChAdOx1 nCoV-19 vaccine by upregulating genes promoting memory T cell responses
by: Nature Publishing Group | **Release Date:** 20 June 2024
Website: Nature | **Publisher:** npj Vaccines

[s183] - https://porcinehealthmanagement.biomedcentral.com/articles/10.1186/s40813-023-00307-z
Author: Carmen Alvárez-Delgado, Ins Ruedas-Torres, Jos M. Sanchez-Carvajal, Feliciano Priego-Capote, Laura Castillo-Peinado, Angela Galan-Relao, Pedro J. Moreno, Esperanza Diaz-Bueno, Benito Lozano-Buenestado, Irene M. Rodriguez-Gomez, Librado Carrasco, Francisco J. Pallares, Jaime Gomez-Laguna
Title: Impact of supplementation with dihydroxylated vitamin D3 on performance parameters and gut health in weaned Iberian piglets under indooroutdoor conditions
by: BMC
Website: Porcine Health Management
Release Date: 2023-06-15
Publisher: BMC

[s184] - https://joe.bioscientifica.com/view/journals/joe/224/3/R107.xml
Title: Immunological role of vitamin D at the maternalfetal interface
Website: Journal of Endocrinology
by: Bioscientifica

[s185] - https://pubmed.ncbi.nlm.nih.gov/31963293/
Author: Adrian F Gombart, Adeline Pierre, Silvia Maggini
Title: A Review of Micronutrients and the Immune System-Working in Harmony to Reduce the Risk of Infection
by: Bayer Consumer Care AG
Website: PubMed
Release Date: 2020-01-16
Publisher: MDPI

[s186] - https://bmcnutr.biomedcentral.com/articles/10.1186/2055-0928-1-7
Author: Steve Simpson Jr, Ingrid van der Mei, Niall Stewart, Leigh Blizzard, Prudence Tettey, Bruce Taylor
Title: Weekly cholecalciferol supplementation results in significant reductions in infection risk among the vitamin D deficient: results from the CIPRIS pilot RCT
by: BMC Nutrition
Website: BMC Nutrition
Release Date: 09 March 2015
Publisher: BioMed Central

[s187] - https://www.ncbi.nlm.nih.gov/pmc/articles/PMC7230749/
Author: Philip C Calder, Anitra C Carr, Adrian F Gombart, Manfred Eggersdorfer
Title: Optimal Nutritional Status for a Well-Functioning Immune System Is an Important Factor to Protect against Viral Infections
by: MDPI
Website: NCBI
Release Date: 2020-04-23
Publisher: MDPI

[s188] - https://www.yalemedicine.org/news/long-covid-treatment-does-your-vitamin-d-level-play-a-role
Author: Kenny Cheng
Title: Long COVID treatment: Does your vitamin D level play a role?
by: Yale Medicine
Website: Yale Medicine
Release Date: April 29, 2024
Publisher: Yale University

[s189] - https://www.ncbi.nlm.nih.gov/geo/query/acc.cgi?acc=GSE86406
Author: Scott JF, Das LM, Ahsanuddin S, Qui Y, Binko A, Traylor ZP, Debanne S, Cooper KD, Boxer R, Lu KQ
Title: Oral vitamin D for the attenuation of sunburn
by: Case Western Reserve University University Hospitals Case Medical Ctr
Website: NCBI
Release Date: Feb 16, 2018

[s190] - https://pure.eur.nl/files/47751761/fimmu-07-00697.pdf
Author: Wendy Dankers, Edgar M. Colin, Jan Piet van Hamburg, Erik Lubberts
Title: Vitamin D in Autoimmunity: Molecular Mechanisms and Therapeutic Potential
by: Erasmus MC, University Medical Center
Website: Frontiers in Immunology
Release Date: 01012017
Publisher: Frontiers Media SA

[s191] - https://www.ncbi.nlm.nih.gov/pmc/articles/PMC8902492/
Author: Matheus Ribeiro Bizuti, Edina Starck, Kimberly Kamila da Silva Fagundes, Josiano Guilherme Puhle, Lucas Medeiros Lima, Natan Rodrigues de Oliveira, Guilherme Vinicio de Sousa Silva, Dbora Tavares Resende e Silva
Title: Influence of exercise and vitamin D on the immune system against Covid-19: an integrative review of current literature
by: Federal University of Fronteira Sul
Website: NCBI
Release Date: 2022-03-08
Publisher: Springer Science+Business Media, LLC, part of Springer Nature

[s192] - https://epag.springeropen.com/articles/10.1186/s43054-022-00135-w
Author: Nevin Sanlier, Merve Guney-Coskun
Title: Vitamin D, the immune system, and its relationship with diseases
by: Egyptian Pediatric Association Gazette
Website: SpringerOpen
Release Date: 17 October 2022

[s193] - https://medlineplus.gov/lab-tests/vitamin-d-test/
Title: Vitamin D Test
Website: MedlinePlus
by: National Library of Medicine

[s194] - https://www.cancer.gov/about-cancer/causes-prevention/risk/diet/vitamin-d-fact-sheet
Title: Vitamin D and Cancer
Release Date: May 9, 2023
Publisher: U.S. Department of Health and Human Services
by: National Cancer Institute
Website: cancer.gov

[s195] - https://www.ncbi.nlm.nih.gov/books/NBK441912/
Author: Krati Chauhan; Mahsa Shahrokhi; Martin R. Huecker
Title: Vitamin D
by: StatPearls Publishing
Website: NCBI Bookshelf
Release Date: 2024 Jan-
Publisher: National Library of Medicine, National Institutes of Health

[s196] - https://www.nature.com/articles/s41430-020-0558-y
Author: Karin Amrein, Mario Scherkl, Magdalena Hoffmann, Stefan Neuwersch-Sommeregger, Markus Kstenberger, Adelina Tmava Berisha, Gennaro Martucci, Stefan Pilz, Oliver Malle
Title: Vitamin D deficiency 2.0: an update on the current status worldwide
Release Date: 20 January 2020
Publisher: European Journal of Clinical Nutrition
Website: Nature

[s197] - https://www.yalemedicine.org/news/vitamin-d-myths-debunked
Author: Colleen Moriarty
by: Yale Medicine
Website: Yale Medicine
Title: Vitamin D Myths D-bunked
Release Date: March 15, 2018

[s198] - https://www.nhs.uk/conditions/vitamins-and-minerals/vitamin-d/
Title: Vitamin D
Release Date: 03 August 2020
by: NHS
Website: NHS

[s199] - https://pubmed.ncbi.nlm.nih.gov/34202578/
Author: Shaun Sabico, Mushira A Enani, Eman Shes hah, Naji J Aljohani, Dara A Aldisi, Naif H Alotaibi, Naemah Alshingetti, Suliman Y Alomar, Abdullah M Alnaami, Osama E Amer, Syed D Hussain, Nasser M Al-Daghri **Title:** Effects of a 2-Week 5000 IU versus 1000 IU Vitamin D3 Supplementation on Recovery of Symptoms in Patients with Mild to Moderate Covid-19: A Randomized Clinical Trial
by: King Saud University **Release Date:** 2021-06-24
Website: pubmed.ncbi.nlm.nih.gov **Publisher:** Nutrients

[s200] - https://pubmed.ncbi.nlm.nih.gov/19101755/
Author: C J Bacon, G D Gamble, A M Horne, M A Scott, I R Reid **Title:** High-dose oral vitamin D3 supplementation in the elderly
Release Date: 2009-08 **Website:** PubMed
Publisher: Osteoporosis International

[s201] - https://www.ncbi.nlm.nih.gov/books/NBK532266/
Author: Omeed Sizar; Swapnil Khare; Amandeep Goy al; Amy Givler **Title:** Vitamin D Deficiency
by: StatPearls Publishing **Release Date:** 2024 Jan-
Website: NCBI Bookshelf **Publisher:** StatPearls Publishing

[s202]
https://www.bluecrossnc.com/content/dam/bcbsnc/pdf/providers/policies-guidelines-codes/policies/commercial/laboratory/vitamin_d_testing.pdf
Title: Vitamin D Testing AHS G2005 **by:** Blue Cross Blue Shield of North Carolina
Release Date: 01012019 **Website:** Blue Cross Blue Shield of North Carolina

[s203] - https://ejim.springeropen.com/articles/10.1186/s43162-024-00330-8
Author: Marwa Ahmed Salah Ahmed, Mohamed Nabil Soliman Atta, Mona Abdel-Latif Aboul-Seoud, Mona Moustafa Tahoun, Sarah Abd El Rahim Rady Abd Allah **Title:** Assessment of vitamin d status among egy ptian covid-19 patients
Release Date: 14 June 2024 **Website:** The Egyptian Journal of Internal Medicine
Publisher: SpringerOpen

[s204] - https://medlineplus.gov/lab-tests/vitamin-d-test/
Title: Vitamin D Test **by:** National Library of Medicine
Website: MedlinePlus

[s205] - https://www.ncbi.nlm.nih.gov/pmc/articles/PMC7282243/
Author: Esin Avci, Suleyman Demir, Diler Aslan, Rukiye Nar, Hande Senol **Title:** Assessment of Abbott Architect 25-OH vitamin D assay in different levels of vitamin D
by: Pamukkale University **Release Date:** 2020-01-10
Website: NCBI **Publisher:** CEONCEES

[s206] - https://pubmed.ncbi.nlm.nih.gov/27834063/
Author: Hyun Jeong Kim, Misuk Ji, Junghan Song, Hee Won Moon, Mina Hur, Yeo Min Yun **Title:** Clinical Utility of Measurement of Vitamin D-Binding Protein and Calculation of Bioavailab le Vitamin D in Assessment of Vitamin D Status
by: Korean Association of Health Promotion **Release Date:** 2017-01
Website: PubMed **Publisher:** Ann Lab Med

[s207] - https://link.springer.com/article/10.1007/s00223-022-00961-5
Author: N. Alonso, S. Zelzer, G. Eibinger, M. He rrmann **Title:** Vitamin D Metabolites: Analytical Challenges and Clinical Relevance
by: Springer **Release Date:** 2022-03-03
Website: SpringerLink **Publisher:** Calcified Tissue International

[s208] - https://www.ncbi.nlm.nih.gov/pmc/articles/PMC2827576/
Author: Ishir Bhan, Sherri-Ann M Burnett-Bowie, Jun Ye, Marcello Tonelli, Ravi Thadhani **Title:** Clinical Measures Identify Vitamin D Def iciency in Dialysis
by: Massachusetts General Hospital, University of Alberta **Release Date:** 2010-03
Website: NCBI **Publisher:** American Society of Nephrology

[s209] - https://medlineplus.gov/lab-tests/vitamin-d-test/
Title: Vitamin D Test **by:** National Library of Medicine
Website: MedlinePlus

[s210] - https://www.ncbi.nlm.nih.gov/books/NBK441912/
Author: Krati Chauhan; Mahsa Shahrokhi; Martin R. Huecker **Title:** Vitamin D
by: StatPearls Publishing **Release Date:** 2024 Jan-
Website: NCBI Bookshelf **Publisher:** National Library of Medicine, National I nstitutes of Health

[s211] - https://www.nature.com/articles/s41430-020-0558-y
Author: Karin Amrein, Mario Scherkl, Magdalena H offmann, Stefan Neuwersch-Sommeregger, M arkus Kstenberger, Adelina Tmava Berisha, Gennaro Martucci, Stefan Pilz, Oliver Malle **Title:** Vitamin D deficiency 2.0: an update on the current status worldwide
by: Nature Publishing Group **Release Date:** 20 January 2020
Website: Nature **Publisher:** European Journal of Clinical Nutrition

[s212] - https://med.virginia.edu/ginutrition/wp-content/uploads/sites/199/2021/06/May-2021-Vitamin-D-Replacement.pdf
Author: Ronak M. Patel, M.D., Lindsay Bazydlo, P h.D., Sue A. Brown, M.D., Alan C. Dalkin, M.D. **Title:** Vitamin D Replacement in Adults: Current Strategies in Clinical Management
by: University of Virginia Health System **Release Date:** May 2021
Website: University of Virginia Health System **Publisher:** Practical Gastroenterology

[s213] - https://secure.arkansasbluecross.com/members/report.aspx?policyNumber=2018006
Title: Coverage Policy Manual **by:** Arkansas Blue Cross Blue Shield
Release Date: February 2018 **Website:** Arkansas Blue Cross Blue Shield

[s214] - https://www2.gov.bc.ca/gov/content/health/practitioner-professional-resources/bc-guidelines/vitamin-d-testing
Title: Vitamin D Testing **by:** Government of British Columbia
Release Date: June 3, 2024 **Website:** Government of British Columbia

[s215]
https://www.bluecrossnc.com/content/dam/bcbsnc/pdf/providers/policies-guidelines-codes/policies/commercial/laboratory/vitamin_d_testing.pdf
Title: Vitamin D Testing AHS G2005 **by:** Blue Cross Blue Shield of North Carolina
Release Date: 01012019 **Website:** Blue Cross Blue Shield of North Carolina

[s216] - https://jhpn.biomedcentral.com/articles/10.1186/s41043-017-0096-y
Author: Sakineh Nouri Saeidlou, Davoud Vahabzadeh, Fariba Babaei, Zakaria Vahabzadeh **Title:** Seasonal variations of vitamin D and its relation to lipid profile in Iranian children and adults
by: Urmia University of Medical Sciences **Release Date:** 2017-05-22
Website: Journal of Health, Population and Nutrition **Publisher:** Springer Nature

[s217] - https://pubmed.ncbi.nlm.nih.gov/22865902/
Author: Adrian D Wood, Karen R Secombes, Frank Tthies, Lorna Aucott, Alison J Black, Alexandra Mavroeidi, William G Simpson, William D Fraser, David M Reid, Helen M Macdonald
Title: Vitamin D3 supplementation has no effect on conventional cardiovascular risk factors: a parallel-group, double-blind, placebo-controlled RCT
Release Date: 2012-08-03
Website: PubMed
Publisher: J Clin Endocrinol Metab

[s218] - https://pubmed.ncbi.nlm.nih.gov/15231008/
Author: Christian Meier, Henning W Woitge, Klaus Witte, Bjrn Lemmer, Markus J Seibel
Title: Supplementation with oral vitamin D3 and calcium during winter prevents seasonal bone loss: a randomized controlled open-label prospective trial
by: ANZAC Research Institute
Release Date: 2004-05-24
Website: PubMed
Publisher: J Bone Miner Res

[s219] - https://www.nature.com/articles/s41598-021-98343-8
Author: Susana Flores-Villalva, Megan B. O'Brien, Cian Reid, Sen Lacey, Stephen V. Gordon, Corwin Nelson, Kieran G. Meade
Title: Low serum vitamin D concentrations in Spring-born dairy calves are associated with elevated peripheral leukocytes
by: Nature Publishing Group
Release Date: 2021-09-23
Website: Nature
Publisher: Scientific Reports

[s220] - https://pghn.org/DOIx.php?id=10.5223/pghn.2021.24.2.207
Author: Jong Woo Won, Seong Kwan Jung, In Ah Jung, Yoon Lee
Title: Seasonal Changes in Vitamin D Levels of Healthy Children in Mid-Latitude, Asian Urban Area
by: The Korean Society of Pediatric Gastroenterology, Hepatology and Nutrition
Release Date: 2021-03-04
Website: Pediatric Gastroenterology, Hepatology Nutrition

[s221] - https://www.nih.gov/news-events/nih-research-matters/low-vitamin-d-levels-associated-colds-flu
Author: William Duval, Ph.D.
Title: Low Vitamin D Levels Associated with Colds and Flu
by: National Institutes of Health
Release Date: March 9, 2009
Website: NIH Research Matters
Publisher: U.S. Department of Health Human Services

[s222] - https://www.ncbi.nlm.nih.gov/books/NBK557876/
Author: Anum Asif; Nauman Farooq
Title: Vitamin D Toxicity
by: StatPearls Publishing
Release Date: 2024 Jan
Website: NCBI Bookshelf
Publisher: StatPearls Publishing

[s223] - https://www.nhs.uk/conditions/vitamins-and-minerals/vitamin-d/
Title: Vitamin D
by: NHS
Release Date: 03 August 2020
Website: NHS

[s224] - https://medlineplus.gov/ency/article/002596.htm
Author: Jesse Borke, MD, CPE, FAAEM, FACEP
Title: Multiple vitamin overdose
by: A.D.A.M., Inc.
Release Date: 07012023
Website: MedlinePlus
Publisher: National Library of Medicine

[s225] - https://article.imrpress.com/journal/IJVNR/94/2/10.1024/0300-9831/a000798/0434350f16f4c5c21f1b3d412be7e2f4.pdf
Author: Zahra Nekoukar, Aliasghar Manouchehri, Zakaria Zakariaei
Title: Accidental vitamin D3 overdose in a young man: A case report and literature of review
Release Date: November 17, 2023
Website: International Journal for Vitamin and Nutrition Research
Publisher: Hogrefe Publishing

[s226] - https://www.ncbi.nlm.nih.gov/books/NBK557876/
Author: Anum Asif; Nauman Farooq
Title: Vitamin D Toxicity
by: StatPearls Publishing
Release Date: 2024 Jan
Website: NCBI Bookshelf
Publisher: StatPearls Publishing

[s227] - https://pubmed.ncbi.nlm.nih.gov/30294301/
Author: Ewa Marcinowska-Suchowierska, Malgorzata Kupisz-Urbanska, Jacek Lukaszkiewicz, Pawel Pludowski, Glenville Jones
Title: Vitamin D Toxicity-A Clinical Perspective
Release Date: 2018-09-20
Website: Front Endocrinol (Lausanne)

[s228] - https://jmedicalcasereports.biomedcentral.com/articles/10.1186/1752-1947-8-74
Author: Rinkesh Kumar Bansal, Pankaj Tyagi, Praveen Sharma, Vikas Singla, Veronica Arora, Naresh Bansal, Ashish Kumar, Anil Arora
Title: Iatrogenic hypervitaminosis D as an unusual cause of persistent vomiting: a case report
by: BioMed Central Ltd
Release Date: 26 February 2014
Website: Journal of Medical Case Reports
Publisher: BioMed Central

[s229] - https://bmcpediatr.biomedcentral.com/articles/10.1186/s12887-020-02240-4
Author: Fariba Farnaghi, Hossein Hassanian-Moghaddam, Nasim Zamani, Narges Gholami, Latif Gachkar, Maryam Hosseini Yazdi
Title: Vitamin D toxicity in a pediatric toxicological referral center; a cross-sectional study from Iran
by: Shahid Beheshti University of Medical Sciences
Release Date: 20 July 2020
Website: BMC Pediatrics
Publisher: Springer Nature

[s230] - https://www.nature.com/articles/s41598-021-87099-w
Author: Thomas Plant-Bordeneuve, Silvia Berardis, Pierre Bastin, Damien Gruson, Laurence Henri, Sophie Gohy
Title: Vitamin D intoxication in patients with cystic fibrosis: report of a single-center cohort
by: Cliniques universitaires Saint-Luc
Release Date: 08 April 2021
Website: Nature
Publisher: Scientific Reports

[s231] - https://www.ncbi.nlm.nih.gov/books/NBK548094/
Title: LiverTox: Clinical and Research Information on Drug-Induced Liver Injury
by: National Institute of Diabetes and Digestive and Kidney Diseases
Release Date: 2012-05-27
Website: NCBI
Publisher: National Library of Medicine

[s232] - https://www.nature.com/articles/s41430-020-0558-y
Author: Karin Amrein, Mario Scherkl, Magdalena Hoffmann, Stefan Neuwersch-Sommeregger, Markus Kstenberger, Adelina Tmava Berisha, Gennaro Martucci, Stefan Pilz, Oliver Malle
Title: Vitamin D deficiency 2.0: an update on the current status worldwide
by: Nature Publishing Group
Release Date: 20 January 2020
Website: nature.com
Publisher: European Journal of Clinical Nutrition

[s233] - https://pubmed.ncbi.nlm.nih.gov/18290725/
Author: Reinhold Vieth
Title: Vitamin D toxicity, policy, and science
Release Date: 2007-12
Website: PubMed
Publisher: J Bone Miner Res

[s234] - https://www.efsa.europa.eu/sites/default/files/2024-05/ul-summary-report.pdf
Title: Overview on Tolerable Upper Intake Levels by:
Release Date: June 2024 Website:
European Food Safety Authority
EFSA

[s235] - https://link.springer.com/article/10.1007/s40520-020-01678-x
Author: Ren Rizzoli Title:
Vitamin D supplementation: upper limit for safety revisited?
Release Date: 28 August 2020 Website: SpringerLink
Publisher: Aging Clinical and Experimental Research

[s236]
https://www.canada.ca/en/health-canada/services/drugs-health-products/drug-products/prescription-drug-list/notices-changes/notice-amendment-vitamin-d.html
Title: Notice: Prescription Drug List (PDL): Vitamin by:
D
Health Canada
Release Date: 2021-02-22 Website: Canada.ca
Publisher: Government of Canada

[s237] - https://ucfhealth.com/our-services/lifestyle-medicine/how-to-flush-vitamin-d-out-of-system/
Title: How to Flush Vitamin D Out of Your System by:
Naturally
UCF Health
Website: ucfhealth.com

[s238] - https://www.ncbi.nlm.nih.gov/books/NBK557876/
Author: Anum Asif; Nauman Farooq Title: Vitamin D Toxicity
by: StatPearls Publishing Release Date: 2024 Jan
Website: NCBI Bookshelf Publisher: StatPearls Publishing

[s239] - https://medlineplus.gov/ency/article/002596.htm
Author: Jesse Borke, MD, CPE, FAAEM, FACEP Title: Multiple vitamin overdose
by: A.D.A.M., Inc. Release Date: 07012023
Website: MedlinePlus Publisher: National Library of Medicine

[s240] - https://pubmed.ncbi.nlm.nih.gov/30294301/
Author: Ewa Marcinowska-Suchowierska, Malgorzata Title: Vitamin D Toxicity-A Clinical Perspective
Kupisz-Urbanska, Jacek Lukaszkiewicz, Pawel
Pludowski, Glenville Jones
Release Date: 2018-09-20 Website: Front Endocrinol (Lausanne)

[s241] - https://www.nhs.uk/conditions/vitamins-and-minerals/vitamin-d/
Title: Vitamin D by: NHS
Release Date: 03 August 2020 Website: NHS

[s242] - https://www.ncbi.nlm.nih.gov/books/NBK548094/
Title: LiverTox: Clinical and Research Information by:
on Drug-Induced Liver Injury
National Institute of Diabetes and Digestive and Kidney Diseases
Release Date: 2012-05-27 Website: NCBI

[s243] - https://www.kidney.org/sites/default/files/Vitamin-D-Supplementation-Patients-With-CKD.pdf
Author: Holly Kramer, MD, MPH; Jeffrey S. Berns, Title: 25-Hydroxyvitamin D Testing and Suppleme
MD; Michael J. Choi, MD; Kevin Martin, ntation in CKD: An NKF-KDOQI Controversi
MD; Michael V. Rocco, MD es Report
by: National Kidney Foundation Release Date: July 28, 2014
Website: Kidney.org Publisher: Elsevier Inc.

[s244] - https://link.springer.com/article/10.1007/s00223-021-00844-1
Author: Marilena Christodoulou, Terence J. Aspray, Title: Vitamin D Supplementation for Patients with
Inez Schoenmakers Chronic Kidney Disease: A Systematic Review
and Meta-analyses of Trials Investigating the
Response to Supplementation and an Overview
of Guidelines
by: Springer Release Date: 2021-04-25
Website: SpringerLink Publisher: Calcified Tissue International

[s245] - https://pubmed.ncbi.nlm.nih.gov/24753153/
Author: Lieke S Kamphuis, Femke Bonte-Mineur, Jan Title: Calcium and vitamin D in sarcoidosis: is
A van Laar, P Martin van Hagen, Paul L van supplementation safe?
Daele
by: Erasmus MC, University Medical Centre Release Date: 2014-11
Website: PubMed Publisher: American Society for Bone and Mineral Re
search

[s246] - https://ern-lung.eu/wp-content/uploads/2020/12/1a.-Guideline-sarcoidosis-diagnosis-ATS-2020.pdf
Author: Elliott D. Crouser, Lisa A. Maier, Kevin C. Title: Diagnosis and Detection of Sarcoidosis: An
Wilson, Catherine A. Bonham, Adam S. Official American Thoracic Society Clinical
Morgenthau, Karen C. Patterson, Eric Abston, Practice Guideline
Richard C. Bernstein, Ron Blankstein, Edward
S. Chen, Daniel A. Culver, Wonder Drake,
Marjolein Drent, Alicia K. Gerke, Michael
Ghobrial, Praveen Govender, Nabeel Hamzeh,
W. Ennis James, Marc A. Judson, Liz Kellerm
eyer, Shandra Knight, Laura L. Koth, Venerino
Poletti, Subha V. Raman, Melissa H. Tukey, G
loria E. Westney, Robert P. Baughman
by: American Thoracic Society Release Date: February 2020
Website: American Thoracic Society Publisher: American Thoracic Society

[s247] - https://www.ncbi.nlm.nih.gov/books/NBK559248/
Author: Hacen Vall; Preeti Patel; Mayur Parmar Title: Teriparatide
by: StatPearls Publishing Release Date: 2024 Jan
Website: NCBI Bookshelf Publisher: National Library of Medicine, National I
nstitutes of Health

[s248] - https://www.hey.nhs.uk/wp/wp-content/uploads/2016/03/vitaminD.pdf
Author: Dr Mo Aye, Consultant Endocrinologist; Dr Title: Prescribing Guideline: Vitamin D: testing and
Marie Miller, Interface Pharmacist replacement
by: Hull and East Riding Prescribing Committee Release Date: Approved: HERPC Sept 2014 Updated: Aug 2
018 Review: Aug 2021
Website: NHS

[s249] - https://pubmed.ncbi.nlm.nih.gov/34847425/
Author: Carla LoPinto-Khoury, Laura Brennan, Scott Title: Impact of carbamazepine on vitamin D levels:
Mintzer A meta-analysis
by: Temple University, Thomas Jefferson Univ Release Date: 2021-11-26
ersity
Website: PubMed Publisher: Elsevier B.V.

[s250] - https://www.e-acnm.org/journal/view.html?doi=10.15747/ACNM.2022.14.1.20

Author:	Jung Won Jung, So Young Park, Hyunah Kim	**Title:**	Drug-Induced Vitamin Deficiency
by:	Sookmyung Women's University	**Release Date:**	June 1, 2022
Website:	Annals of Clinical Nutrition and Metabolism	**Publisher:**	The Korean Society of Surgical Metabolism and Nutrition and The Korean Society for Parenteral and Enteral Nutrition

[s251] - https://www.nature.com/articles/sc2016131

Author:	J Lamarche, G Mailhot	**Title:**	Vitamin D and spinal cord injury: should we care?
by:	Nature Publishing Group	**Release Date:**	20 September 2016
Website:	nature.com	**Publisher:**	Nature Publishing Group

Image Sources

Information about all following images
None of the images were modified, only the resolution was adjusted.
All images retain their original license.
Despite careful review, the accuracy and attribution of images cannot be guaranteed.
All images used were used in accordance with their respective licence terms.
In the eBook version, the images have been compiled into numbered collages.
All images were finally retrieved and verified 2024-12-20.

Used Licenses

CC0	http://creativecommons.org/publicdomain/zero/1.0/deed.en
CC BY 4.0	https://creativecommons.org/licenses/by/4.0
CC BY 2.0	https://creativecommons.org/licenses/by/2.0

Image Credits

[i1] - 001_001_001_image_7dehydrocholesterin.jpeg
https://upload.wikimedia.org/wikipedia/commons/a/a0/7-Dehydrocholesterol_molecule_spacefill.png
Date: 2011-08-04   by: Jynto
License: CC0 (http:creativecommons.orgpublicdomainzero1.0deed.en)

[i2] - 001_002_003_image_vitamin_d.jpeg
https://upload.wikimedia.org/wikipedia/commons/b/b4/Cholecalciferol-vitamin-D3-from-xtal-3D-sticks.png
Date: 2009-03-23   by: Benjah-bmm27
Artist: Ben Mills   License: Public domain

[i3] - 001_003_002_image_lachs.jpeg
https://upload.wikimedia.org/wikipedia/commons/1/1e/Pink_salmon_FWS.jpg
Date: 2001   by: Citron
Artist: Timothy Knepp   License: Public domain

[i4] - 001_003_002_image_muesli.jpeg
https://upload.wikimedia.org/wikipedia/commons/2/28/Chocolate-muesli.jpg
Date: 2016-05-22   by: MartinThoma
License: CC0 (http:creativecommons.orgpublicdomainzero1.0deed.en)

[i5] - 001_003_002_image_pflanzendrink.jpeg
https://upload.wikimedia.org/wikipedia/commons/1/13/Barley_milk.jpg
Date: 2023-04-09   by: Mx. Granger
License: CC0 (http:creativecommons.orgpublicdomainzero1.0deed.en)

[i6] - 001_003_003_image_cerealien.jpeg
https://upload.wikimedia.org/wikipedia/commons/5/56/Cereal-Fruity-Pebbles.jpg
Date: 2014-11-19   by: Evan-Amos
License: Public domain

[i7] - 001_003_004_image_kapseln.jpeg
https://upload.wikimedia.org/wikipedia/commons/7/75/Arranging_capsules.jpg
Date: 2023-11-15   by: M Joko Apriyo Putro
License: CC BY 4.0 (https:creativecommons.orglicensesby4.0)

[i8] - 001_003_005_image_vitamin_dbindendes_protein.jpeg
https://upload.wikimedia.org/wikipedia/commons/f/f5/PDB_fkxp_EBI.jpg
Date: 2009-03-11   by: DonabelSDSU.bot
Artist: European Bioinformatics Institute   License: Public domain

[i9] - 002_001_001_image_supplementierung.jpeg
https://upload.wikimedia.org/wikipedia/commons/5/52/Quercetin_Supplement_Capsules_-_53398952524.jpg
Date: 2023-12-15   by: Longevityfaq
Artist: ben_hoffman2003   License: CC BY 2.0 (https:creativecommons.orglicensesby2.0)

[i10] - 003_001_001_image_calcium.jpeg
https://upload.wikimedia.org/wikipedia/commons/d/db/Naturalis_Biodiversity_Center_-_Gypsum_-_mineral.jpg
Date: 2014-08-06   by: Hansmuller
Artist: Naturalis Biodiversity Center   License: CC0 (http:creativecommons.orgpublicdomainzero1.0deed.en)

[i11] - 003_001_001_image_rankl.jpeg
https://upload.wikimedia.org/wikipedia/commons/3/34/PDB_1s55_EBI.jpg
Date: 2009-02-20   **by:** DonabelSDSU.bot
Artist: European Bioinformatics Institute   **License:** Public domain

[i12] - 004_002_002_image_kreatinin.jpeg
https://upload.wikimedia.org/wikipedia/commons/3/33/Creatinine-amino-tautomer-3D-vdW.png
Date: 2021-09-02   **by:** Hoahocphantu
License: Public domain

[i13] - 004_003_003_image_urolithiasis.jpeg
https://upload.wikimedia.org/wikipedia/commons/1/1b/Kidney_stone_4mm_05.jpg
Date: unknown   **by:** Eduardschnack
Artist: Jacek Proszyk   **License:** CC0   (http:creativecommons.orgpublicdomai
                                                        nzero1.0deed.en)

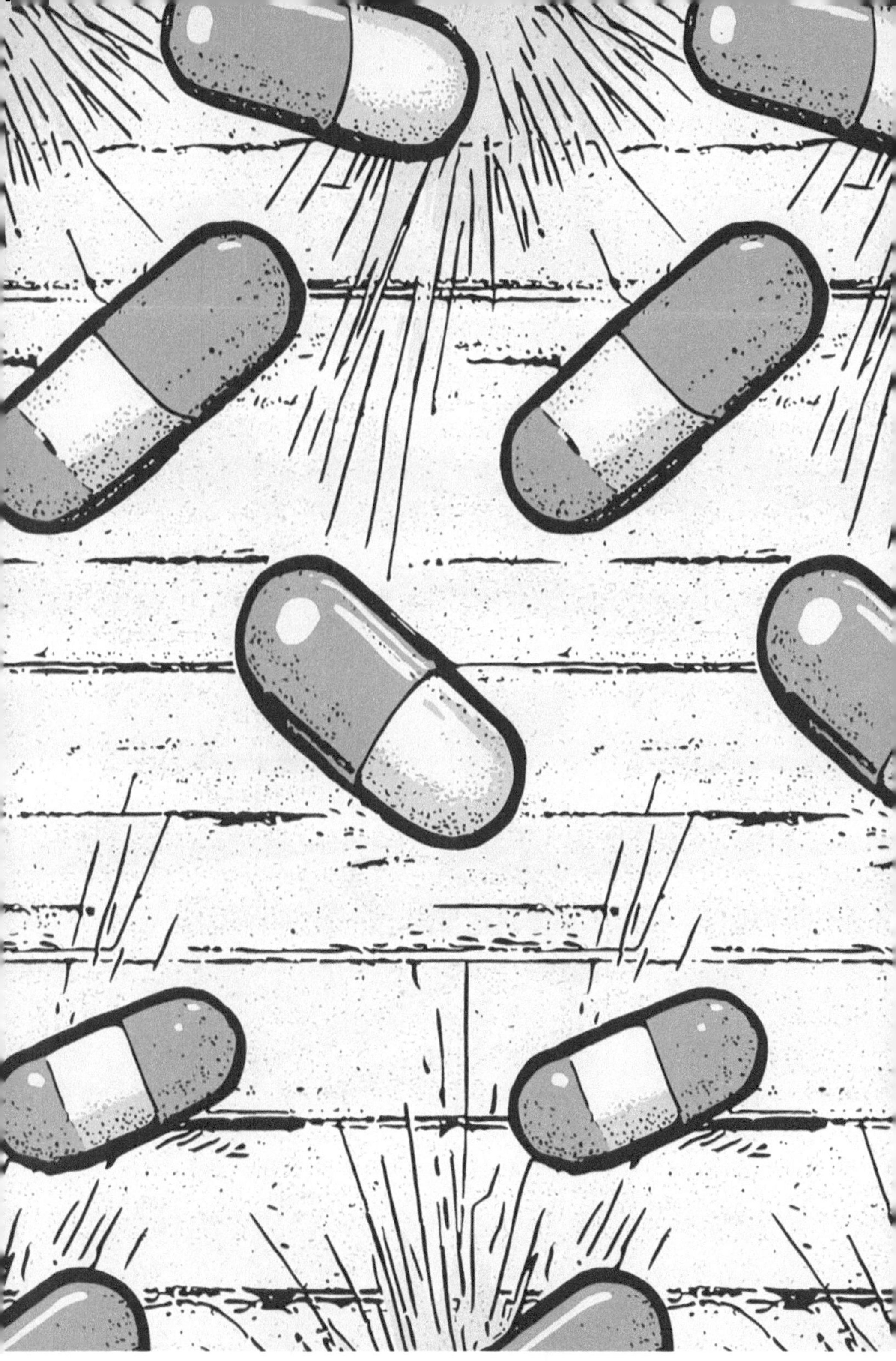

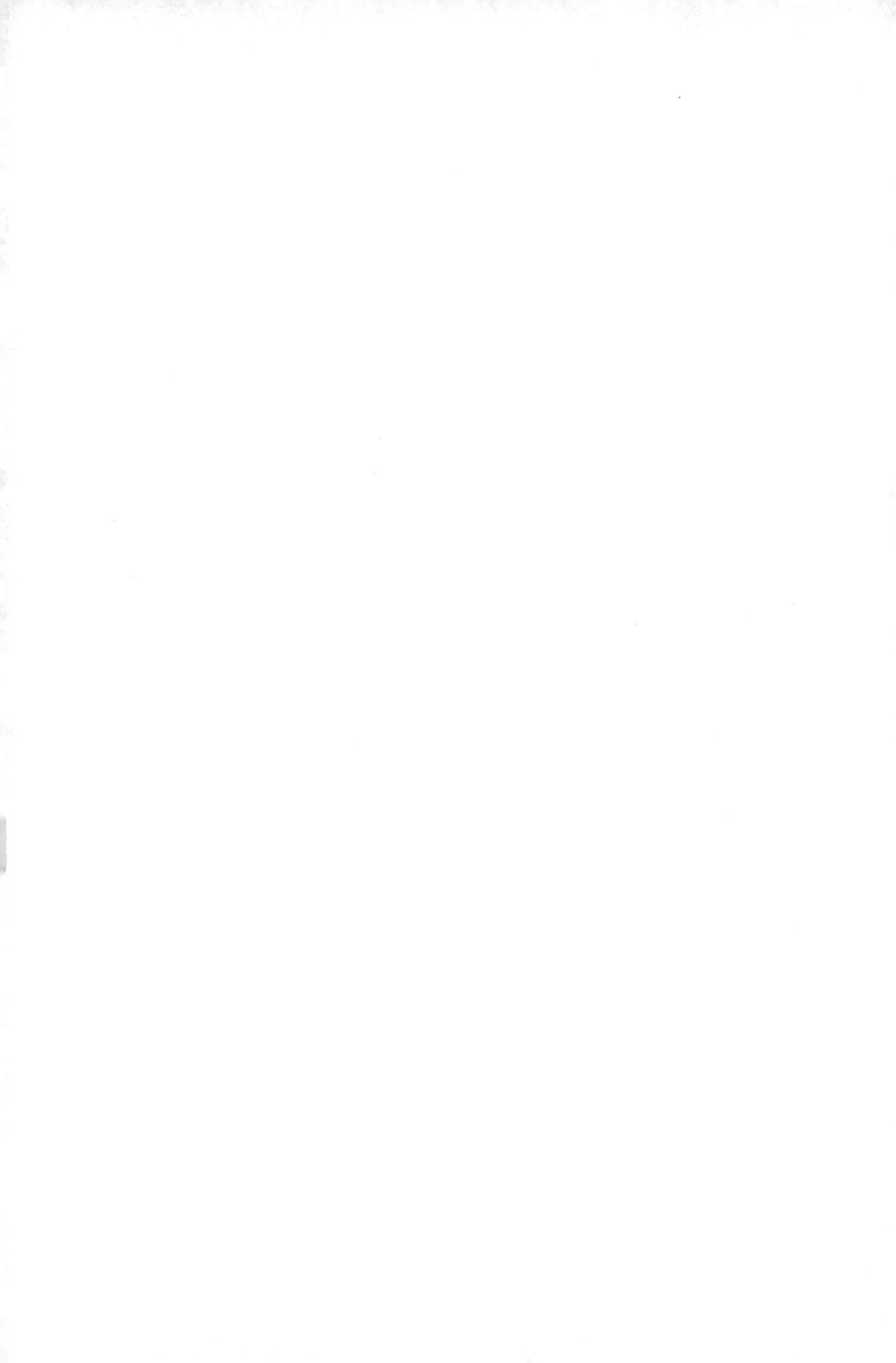

www.ingramcontent.com/pod-product-compliance
Lightning Source LLC
LaVergne TN
LVHW042112190726
843493LV00006B/1453